—WHY—
WEIGHT?

HOW TO BE HAPPY EVERY DAY
WHATEVER THE SCALES SAY

HEIDI STRICKLAND-CLARK

RƎTHINK PRESS

First published in Great Britain 2017 by Rethink
Press (www.rethinkpress.com)

Cover image © Shutterstock / Nikita TV
Author photo © Dale Strickland-Clark
Illustrations © Heidi Sandford

Each copy of this book sold gives the gift of sight to an Indonesian
who cannot afford a pair of glasses. Thank you for seeing
things differently and helping to make a huge difference.

We are a proud partner of B1G1 – a Social Enterprise with a
mission to create a world that's full of giving. www.b1g1.com

Contents

CONTENTS

CONTENTS

To anyone who has ever used their weight as
a stick with which to beat themselves.

Introduction

The world does not need another diet book.

If you go to Amazon and search weight loss, you will find over 65,434 books all designed to help you lose weight.

This isn't one of them.

Every morning, many women get out of bed and weigh themselves. They allow the flashing display or wavering dial to dictate how they feel and behave that day. It's become ingrained in what they do and is the indicator for what they'll wear, how they'll react to their partner and children, and how they'll do their job.

My goal for this book is to show you that you don't need to

step on the scales to work out how to feel or prove how good you are. I am going to share with you the ways to be happier, more relaxed and healthier in mind and body without the validation of the scales.

Since 2001 I've worked with women who want to feel happy, rather than having guilt over food, and to eat to live, not live to eat (with all the worry that goes with it).

Chances are you have been on diets for years. Your life may be full, but you feel like something is missing. It's been said that the Universe abhors a void, so if something is missing, the void needs to be filled. For many people, it's filled with food.

Keeping this need to eat under control then leads to the next step, which is the daily, sometimes hourly, checking of weight. It becomes an obsessive response to a problem that hasn't really been addressed, which is not that you're 'rubbish with food' – a desperate plea I often hear from women who don't know what to do next. In fact, I'll be so bold as to say that the problem has nothing to do with food.

The problem is that these women have not found out what is missing; they've not discovered what is sitting in their soul, making them feel unhappy. They have to address this problem in order to stop the persistent need to feel better about their relationship with food.

Who is this book for? It is for you if you can relate to one or more of the following:

- Before you've even got out of bed in the morning, you're thinking about your tummy/bum/legs

- You weigh yourself as soon as you get up

- You weigh yourself before you go to bed

- You'll move the scales or your body position to get the weight you want

- The number on the scales determines your mood, the clothes you wear, your day

- You are frequently thinking about your weight and what to eat to 'be good'

- You are constantly looking for new ways to lose weight

- You feel you need to treat yourself with food each day

- You are tired all the time

- You have been on a diet for most of your adult life

- You think that if you could just lose weight, you'd be happier

- Your weight was an issue within your family when you were a child

- You feel overwhelmed with information and don't know what to do any more

- You've thought at times that you're 'rubbish with food'.

This is not some airy-fairy book. This is not a diet. I want to show you how to get out of the cycle of obsessing over weight and food. It will take some time, but it has worked for me and many other women. It can be as liberating for you as it was for us.

Are you ready to make some changes?

There is no one way for all humans to be slim, happy, healthy and content. We are unique bundles of muscles, organs, metabolic types, lifestyle choices, experiences, likes, dislikes and beliefs. I want you to find your own way, and I'll show you how to do that.

My step by step plan will gently guide you, and the 100 Day Challenge at the back of the book takes you through a process that you can do over 100 days. I'll also share my story and the stories of clients I have helped.

I believe we are never 'done'; we're always changing, from the challenges we face to the experiences we have. So evolve, make your life your own and bloom.

Laura's story

Before we move into the nitty-gritty, I want to share something that our daughter taught me when she was three.

I was a young mum by today's standards. I had Laura at twenty-three and Sophie at twenty-four, and my childbearing days were over before some people had even considered a career. I really wanted a family, but I was young and naïve, and just assumed that my children would be perfect.

When she was three, Laura had her standard community nurse visit which involved an eye test. It transpired that Laura's eyesight was not perfect and further investigation was needed. We ended up having several ophthalmic appointments in the hospital before receiving a prescription to get her some glasses.

Even that was a drawn-out affair. Due to the unusual nature of Laura's eyesight, we had a limited range of frames to choose from, and once we'd chosen, it took ten days before the glasses arrived back in the shop.

We were eventually called in to collect Laura's glasses. I can remember the day so clearly. She and I trundled off to see the optician and waited whilst they fitted the glasses to her face. After paying for the glasses, I took Laura's hand and we walked out into the shopping precinct.

We'd not been walking long when I became aware that she was walking in a strange way, lifting her knees high as though she had to keep stepping over logs.

'Are you alright?' I asked.

'Mummy, my feet are so big and the ground is so close.'

I realised that for three years, Laura's perception of the world had been through wonky eyes. But she had known no different. She had functioned fine. She was walking, talking, learning and watching television in the only way she knew. But as soon as we gave her the ability to see fully and take in the full picture of her surroundings, she had to re-learn what was normal and possible and true to her.

This is what I want for you. I want to give you a new pair of glasses. What you thought to be true for you doesn't necessarily have to be so. With a new outlook, you can see beyond the scales and learn how to have a happy day, every day.

My story

My life has been about size, weight and diets since I was about ten or eleven.

I was the tallest girl in school. So much so that when I went into the secretary's office at junior school, people thought I was one of the mums.

Because I was tall, people would say things like 'Aren't you big?' or 'when did you get so large?' They meant it kindly, but my young brain heard *big* without realising they meant *tall*, not *fat*.

And whilst I wasn't fat, I still felt out of place amongst my peers. I had a bust at the age of ten that many women would have been pleased with, and was wearing a bra in junior school because I needed one, not because I wanted to be 'grown up'. What I really wanted was to fit in, and fitting in at that time meant not wearing a bra. It drew attention to me, and I went into my pre-teens as quite a self-conscious person.

I had always been a fairly good and keen swimmer. After

winning a race in a school gala at the age of eleven, I was encouraged by my mum to join the local swimming club. My teenage years were established as I spent most days swimming lengths.

But there was one moment I particularly remember. I was pulled over by my swimming coach, who told me that if I was going to be any good as a swimmer, I would need to lose weight. I was fourteen, 5 ft 10 inches and had a hefty chest for a young girl, but I wasn't fat. I was a size 10 and well proportioned. But the seed was sown.

I wasn't good enough. I was too fat.

I stopped swimming when I was fifteen due to a knee injury. From swimming over ten hours a week, I became completely inactive, and over a couple of years I gained two stone. By the time I entered sixth form, I was the heaviest I'd ever been.

I don't remember being really unhappy with this, but I do remember thinking about it a lot. I weighed myself each day and became more and more lethargic and lacking in motivation, to the point where I wasn't going into lessons.

My dad referred me to see a consultant at the hospital who, after examining me, said, 'There's nothing wrong with you, you're just overweight.'

This comment after years of self-talk and external sources telling me I wasn't the right weight pushed me to start a twenty-two-year obsession with dieting, exercise and weighing. It sucked the life out of me. Everything I did was driven by food – 'What can I eat?'; 'When can I eat?'; 'Will I be able to eat?'; 'I can't eat that!'; 'What will they think if I eat that?' – and I fell out of love with myself very quickly.

At the age of forty, I realised that my happiness stemmed not from my food, nor my shape, nor my relationships, but from me. I realised that I was fully responsible for my life, my challenges and reactions, and that if I was going to get what I wanted, I would have to find a way to do it myself, and like myself in the process.

...what's wrong is always available. But so is what's right.

TONY ROBBINS

Realising this changed my life. Since then, I've worked on me and got myself to a point where life is good. I don't know how much I weighed this morning, yesterday morning or last week. I eat good food, I have a drink when I want to, I wear clothes that fit and I am happy with my life and how I show up in it.

This is what I want for you.

Put your new glasses on, take my hand. We're going for a walk.

Before we go any further, I'd like you to make sure you have a notebook or a journal so that you can note things down as we go along. This will make referencing your answers to the various exercises easier, and you can also use it to write down ideas and revelations. I read a line once that said, 'Ideas are like eels. If you don't grab hold of them, they slip away.'

PART ONE

Ask and Analyse

Chapter One

Why Ask Questions?

Insanity: doing the same thing over and over
again and expecting different results.

ALBERT EINSTEIN

Chances are that if you've been on the dieting merry-go-round for a few years, you've tried a lot of stuff. You may have considered meal replacements, slimming clubs, exercise, fat melting wraps, fat blocker tablets, smaller clothes to incentivise you, bigger clothes to make you look smaller. And you've probably tried some of these more than once. But the results haven't stuck.

Diets do work when you do them properly, but if they are quick fixes – like meal replacements or fat melting wraps – as soon as you stop doing them, you'll be back to where you were. And that's not because you've failed or been stupid. It's because it wasn't a sustainable, long-term solution. Let's face it, who really wants to eat powdered soup?

You may think that you're always overweight because your clothes are too tight. But if you keep buying clothes that you'll 'slim into', you are always going to feel a bit too big and uncomfortable. It's a constant reminder that the waistband is pinching. It's an ever present nagging that you're 'not good enough'.

The first part of our process is to ask yourself questions. Lots of them. I'll help you get started, but chances are you'll soon be able to come up with questions of your own.

Please take some time to read this exercise and work on it over a few days. I want it to sow some seeds in your mind and get you questioning why you do what you do, then delve deeper into where this comes from and uncover buried beliefs about yourself that you may not know you have.

Imagine you are a super sleuth who does not accept the first answer as the truth. It may be a superficial truth, but go deeper and make each question multi-layered. This is something that I've done a lot with my clients and myself, and it can, on occasion, bring up some emotion. Please don't be surprised if it does for you.

What questions do I need to ask?

It's wise to assume that Einstein knew what he was talking

about, so if you're going to ask yourself questions, it would be a good idea to ask some new ones and listen to the answers. Questions that have a negative or critical feel will only put you on edge. Imagine that your boss or partner were asking you the questions. I'm sure you'd soon get a bit prickly if they were fault-finding in their approach.

Choose kind questions which you can honestly answer in a way that gives you some positive insight. For example, 'What do I want to change about my eating habits?' is kinder than 'Why am I such a greedy pig?' Following a good question with an honest answer will lead you to ask another question, which will get you closer and closer to the real truth behind your actions. When you have the answer to 'What do I want to change about my eating habits?' you can then ask, 'Why is this important to me?' And when you get that answer, you can ask the same question again.

Digging deeper and deeper will help you to see that what you thought was the problem isn't in fact related.

Here are some questions to get you started.

Health:

- How would I like my health to be in five, ten, fifteen, twenty years' time?

- What's important to me about my health?

- How have I already looked after my health well?

- When was I my healthiest?

- How was health or wellness viewed by my parents when I was a child?

- How would being healthier improve my current life?

Fitness:

- How would I like my fitness to be in five, ten, fifteen, twenty years' time?

- What does being fit mean to me?

- Have I ever been as fit as I think I want to be?

- When was I my fittest?

- What did my parents teach me about fitness?

- How would being fitter improve my current life?

Finances:

- What are my financial goals for five, ten, fifteen, twenty years' time?

- What is important to me about my personal finances?

- When did I have my best financial habits in place?

- What would having my finances sorted do to improve my current life?

Relationships:

- Am I happy with my relationships?

- How would I like to improve the quality of my relationships?

- Whom do I need to improve my relationship with first?

- How would my life be different if my relationships were improved?

This is just a starter for your questioning process. See what else comes up for you when you let your mind ponder over the answers.

You've probably spotted that I've included topics beyond weight, health and fitness in the examples. This is because I believe that the core problem around unhappiness with weight and size is never really weight or size. There is something else out of kilter in your life that hasn't been addressed and, until it is, food and not looking after yourself have become the answer to dealing with it.

As soon as you can identify that, for example, your finances are all over the place and it's making you feel anxious so you eat, or an argument you had with your brother is causing you to stay awake at night, which means that you are tired during the day so you eat badly, you'll know where to focus your attention to fix the problems.

If you're still not sure that this is true and you think food really is the issue, consider when you were last having a great time doing something. It may have been with your family on holiday or reading a great book or head down on a project that you loved at work. Chances are food didn't feature that much as you were fully engaged and happy.

7

You may want to start with one area of your life that appears to be causing you the most unhappiness, or you can address all of them. Looking at a wide aspect of your life will give you a better chance of seeing where some work needs to be done. It's quite common for people to tell me that for years they've been blaming their mother for some aspect of their life, yet when they get to this step and start asking questions, they realise it may actually have been their dad or sister. This completely changes how they view things.

Remember as you go through the exercise to take note of what you say in your answers. Sometimes an answer will appear quickly and surprise you. You may dismiss it as rubbish, but these are probably the answers you need to listen to the most. The ones that come unconsidered and challenge your beliefs about yourself are the ones that your intuition is providing.

Answers

Getting your answers may take some time. It's not something to rush. It's taken many years of programming from you, your parents, your colleagues, bosses and the media to get you to the way you feel now. So taking some time to dig deep and listen to what you come up with will be worth it.

Start to understand yourself better so that you can assess why you've behaved the way you have up to now and be motivated and pleased to make some changes because you understand where they have come from. However, this doesn't mean that you'll skip off into the sunset, never worrying about your weight again. Sorry. Something may come up in the future that challenges a hidden idea you've not yet experienced. We are works in progress, and if we can accept that and treat ourselves as such, life becomes infinitely easier and calmer and kinder.

As you go through the multi-layered process of questions, questions, questions, see if there is a pattern. Is there a root to the problem? Is it one person? Is it one small part of your life that you have grown out of all proportion? Is what you're longing to have again a rosy image of something that never really happened?

There are no right or wrong answers here. I just want you to understand the story of your life better so you can author it in a happier way from now onwards.

As you drill down, you'll get to a point where you can go no deeper. This means you've made it – the Golden Nugget of what's causing your unhappiness. The answer is likely to be something along the lines of 'I'm not good enough', 'I'm scared', 'I'm not lovable' or 'I'm not a nice enough person.'

Take a deep breath, look at the answers you've written, and then ask yourself, 'Is this really true?' If you told your closest friend or partner this deepest, darkest worry about yourself, how would they answer that question?

Put your new specs on and sit with that a while.

Chapter Two

The Impact of Values and Beliefs

Before I started my own self-development journey, I bumbled through life struggling with repeating patterns of behaviour that both challenged and frustrated me. I didn't know why they happened and thought it was normal.

When I worked on myself more, I learned how important the values and beliefs we have about ourselves are. I went to workshops that introduced the concept and read about it in self-help books, and started to see where some of the ideas I had about myself had come from.

It was an exciting time as I realised that I had a choice as to whether to deal with them or live with them.

The full topic of values and beliefs is too big for this book to go into. There are many authors in the market who help you to work on this, from Tony Robbins to Louise Hay to Deepak Chopra. If you really want to break through a repeating pattern of behaviour that is sabotaging you then these are good people to refer to, and you can make use of the Resources section at the back of the book.

We all have values and beliefs about ourselves that were imprinted on us by the people who looked after us when we were young. Their own values and beliefs were probably imprinted on them by their parents too. It's like a relay race with each generation passing on the baton to the next.

Unfortunately, this family lore isn't always useful, positive or true, and our perceptions about who we are, how we behave and what we do can become skewed. If you practise a negative belief for long enough, you'll soon believe it to be true and behave in that way regardless.

One of my clients told me that her mother used to take her to Weight Watchers sessions when she was nine years old. This in itself seems quite a significant thing to do with a child, but after the session her mum would then buy her a cake. This really confused, and now amazes, my client. She also has memories of being called 'Fat-Jane' by her family when she was little. It's not surprising that someone thinks they're fat, even when they're not, when this amount of programming has been set from an early age.

Identifying your values and beliefs is a very useful exercise. When we work within the realms of our personal values, life feels harmonious and happy. If our personal values are challenged then we can feel compromised, discordant and unhappy.

Here's one of my own examples.

One of my personal values is to do a great job. Another is to have financial stability. A few years ago I was approached to do some coaching for a company to support their clients. The pay was good and would supplement my income from my business, so my interest was piqued.

However, I soon found that I was not going to be able to keep up with the company's value of keeping its clients happy. I couldn't do a job to the standard required without my own business suffering. My values around doing a good job for both the company and my own clients were challenged and I felt very uncomfortable.

Within four months, I decided to move on and focus on my clients. I learned that even though financial stability is important to me, it's not as important as doing a great job, and my hierarchy of values appeared.

Building your own hierarchy of values is a really useful idea. Find out where you sit around the areas of your life that you are currently struggling with and what makes you tick smoothly each day.

You can do values work at a high level; they apply across the board, regardless of the area of your life you are thinking about. Your values may be things like fairness, honesty, work ethic, success, kindness, risk taking, supporting, teaching, punctuality... Search for any list of values on the internet and it'll be vast.

When I work with clients around their health and fitness, I like to discover their values in that specific area first to see what they believe and where some of their disconnect comes from. When you understand where your ideas and beliefs about health, fitness, weight and size come from, it can open up your mind to understanding why you may seem to be in the same place as you were years ago.

One of my clients unravelled a memory. Her mother had a belief that if you weren't under ten stone and wearing a size twelve or smaller, then you were 'fat' or 'overweight' and basically not good enough. When my client was a child, her mother would weigh herself every day along with a running commentary about clothes sizing.

When she grew and left home, my client would come home to visit the family at weekends. Her mum would frequently come up behind her and flip out the label from the back of her sweater to check what size she was wearing. If it wasn't a twelve or under, a 'well you know what that means' look or conversation would follow. Even as my client became fitter and healthier, her belief around numbers stayed obsessive as this imprint from her mother stuck for many years. It wasn't until we did the values and beliefs work that she realised she could move on.

She told me, 'I feel like I've turned a page in my book and have a firm grip on the pen, writing my story how I want it to be.'

Discovering your beliefs

Our next exercise may take a little time, but it's worth doing. You may find yourself subconsciously working on it for days after starting. There are some beliefs around weight and happiness that have appeared like a lightbulb to me many years after the first time I addressed them.

You can capture this information in many ways. There is no right way; it's really what works best for you. As there is no such thing as perfect, so no need to aim for it. But you do need to start, so find your way and use it. If it's not working, choose another.

You can:

- Use your journal and write the information down
- Use a large piece of paper and randomly write all over it as your brain unpacks its contents
- Record yourself speaking into a voice recorder on your mobile phone, which may seem a bit weird, but it's a great way of letting your brain work without having to wait for your hand to catch up
- Use word association to spark the imagination
- Use coloured pens
- Use pictures, photographs, magazine images.

Choose the heading to reflect the area of your life that you want to focus on, for example, health, wellness, fitness, weight management, happiness. Just make sure it's something that resonates with you. Then get as many ideas around this topic out of your head and on to a page or voice app as quickly as you can. The ideas can be positive, negative or downright incorrect. They can be something you learned from your parents, something your sister shouted at you or something an ex-lover said. It can be what you believe, what you've heard, or something you read once in *Cosmopolitan*.

Here's an example.

Health, fitness and losing weight. Ideas/beliefs:

- If you're fat, you're stupid
- Fat people can't get a job
- You need to eat low fat foods to be healthy
- Exercising every day is bad for you
- You'll get bad knees if you run
- The only way to lose weight is to count calories
- You must be size ten or smaller, ten stone or lighter
- One won't hurt
- You can treat yourself
- You can eat all you want as long as it's healthy
- My friend lost weight on the Atkins/Dukan/South Beach/5:2/LighterLife Diet so I can too
- No carbs 'til Marbs

- If I don't lose 2 lbs a week I am a failure
- You can diet in the week and have a treat at the weekend
- If your legs rub together it's time to lose weight
- Green tea makes you skinny
- Avocado is full of fat
- Lifting weights makes you muscular and bulky
- It's not ladylike to sweat, grunt, workout to the point of exhaustion
- Overweight people are unhappy/happy/depressed/unlovable/poor parents
- Cutting calories slows your metabolism
- A moment on the lips, a lifetime on the hips
- Clear your plate, there are children in Africa starving.

I'm sure you get the idea. Write it all down. Everything that you believe about the heading you've written.

As you look at the mass of words in front of you, does it strike you that it is the contents of your mind? These words are the ones that you say to yourself each day as you contemplate whether you are going to exercise, what to eat and how to behave. Noisy, isn't it?

The next part of the exercise is to read through each belief to see if you know where it stems from originally. If you can pinpoint the moment you heard it for the first time, even better. Then ask yourself, 'Do I believe this? Is this true?'

If the belief conjures up a vivid memory of an emotional scene, then I am going to suggest you sit with that memory. Look at it as a spectator and see what really went on. Is your memory correct? Was it gossip? Were you young and it was childish name calling?

Was it a spiteful exchange from someone who could have dealt with it better? Was it a parent using a belief system they came by innocently and with no better knowledge? Did it even happen at all or have you merged things you've heard with a memory and blended it into a story that you're using to slow down your progress to happiness?

When I was ten, I went on a school trip. I was sitting on top of a bunk bed with my knees on the on the edge of the bed as my legs dangled down. I can clearly remember my best mate saying, without any malice, 'Aren't your knees big?' It stuck with me for years that I had big knees.

I reminded her of it when we were in our thirties, and she had no memory of saying it at all. Whereas I'd carried it around with me for a ridiculous number of years, thinking it to be true, worrying that my knees were indeed big and making decisions on clothes based around one quick, off-the-cuff comment.

Be honest. Find out where each belief comes from. Ask whether it is true. And question if you still need it in your noddle at all.

Discovering your values

We're now going to do a similar exercise around values. These are the principles that are true to you. When these are in place and you work with them, your life will be calm and peaceful and rewarding. If you work outside of them then you struggle, feel compromised and unhappy. If you like, you can think of them as your rules.

Use the same method as before – word association or word clouds or mind mapping or brain dumping – to capture your information, but this time you are going to use values as the topic you're assessing. Get as many ideas as you have around this topic on to the page as quickly as you can. You need at least ten.

Here's a mixed example to give you some ideas.

Values: health, fitness and losing weight:

- All my food should be cooked from fresh
- My children need a hot meal each day
- I only allow myself one barista coffee a day/week
- I won't buy food out when I have it at home
- Throwing food away is wasteful
- I drink alcohol Friday and Saturday only
- I believe in five portions of fruit and veg a day
- I like to eat cheaply regardless of quality

- I only eat organic

- I want time to exercise for me and then separately with my family

- Exercise is my me time

- I value the quality of my weight loss efforts on how quickly I lose it.

Once you've done this, I want you to put the values in the best order you can. You may want to choose the most important five first; you may want to ask yourself, 'Could I do without this value but not this value?' as a way to identify which to place where. You are looking for a list where the top five values are pretty much non-negotiable and the other five may be more flexible.

So from my list, we may have something that looks like this:

1. All my meals are cooked from fresh

2. My children need a hot meal each day

3. Throwing food away is wasteful

4. I like to eat organic

5. I believe in five portions of fruit and veg a day.

Reorder if necessary and work it through so that you get a hierarchical list of values around food, or health, or whatever topic you're working on, that makes sense to you.

Knowing what's important to you around how you function

will make it easier when it comes to looking after yourself and your family and making decisions. It allows you to know in advance whether not eating organic foods or not giving your children a hot meal is going to throw you out of whack, and why. When we don't work within our values, we feel edgy.

When I did this exercise with a group of ten women, the results were very different, but true for each of them. For some, cooking from scratch every day was a primary value; for others, having a vegetable with each dinner was something they had to achieve. Some wanted to shop once a week, whilst others wanted to shop daily.

There's not a right or wrong answer here, but as you start thinking about what makes your life calmer, it can smooth the decision-making process when life gets a bit stressful. You can ask yourself, 'Does this meet my values? Will this make me feel good?' So please take some time to define your personal values around the things that occupy your mind the most.

If you seem to be constantly worrying about your weight, work on weight, size and self-image values. If you seem to be constantly worrying about your job, spend some time on your career and work values. If you stress about not spending enough time with your family or friends, then focus on these areas first.

Chapter Three

The Chattering Mind

Have you noticed the constant conversation you have with yourself?

We all do it whether we're happy with our lot or not. It's human nature to be questioning, working out what's next and assessing our environment. But people who are happy every day have one way of talking to themselves and people who are less happy or pessimistic tend to have another way.

Before I started my own journey of self-discovery, I was a worrier and a glass-half-empty kind of person. I wasn't really unhappy, but there were ways that I used to attempt to make me feel better each day which were more like Russian Roulette in their outcome.

See if any of these are familiar:

- I would weigh myself each day

- I would weigh myself the day after a particularly large intake of comfort food

- I would eat too much to take away the boredom or stress I felt

- I would drink too much too often on the reckoning that it was a treat

- I'd watch the news each night to feel engaged with what was going on, but go to bed feeling miserable because it was always depressing

- I'd work too hard

- I'd take on more work to earn more

- I'd feel hard done by for working so much

- I'd feel guilty for not being there for my children because I was always working

- I'd justify things I wasn't proud of (didn't meet my values)

- I'd convince myself that life was tough and I was destined to be miserable.

All the time I'd be having an internal chatter: 'Well that's not very good, is it?'; 'If you eat that, you'll be really disappointed. Yeah, but I can start tomorrow/run it off/eat less for dinner'; 'I work so hard, life is tough'; 'You're too fat – sort yourself out'; 'Who do you think you are? You can't do that'. I didn't realise I was doing it. I had no idea that my mindset was so negative; that this constant, noisy babbling in my ear narrated my day. My whole demeanour was affected by it.

I saw people who seemed to have it all and apparently did better than I did, and I thought I should work harder, learn more, do more. But this pulled against my values about how much time I spent with my family. And so I was in a dilemma about how to get out of the swirling waters of indecision.

I don't think I even knew that there was another way.

One Sunday afternoon in August of 2012 I came across a blog post entitled something along the lines of 'How To Have An Awesome Start To Your Day Every Day'. It got my interest and I read it. There was a list of top tips in the blog, and one of the points referred to an audio download by the American motivational speaker Tony Robbins. This audio was 90 minutes long.

Although my inner chatter said, 'You don't have enough time', I listened to the audio and was hooked. I'd not heard Tony Robbins speak before, but was semi-aware of him. His deep, raspy, emotive voice had me completely rapt as I listened to how he starts his day with his 'Hour of Power'. There were tips for being active and breathing in a certain way, but there was also a section on the words we say to ourselves and how changing them will change how our day runs.

He said one thing in that 90-minute audio that has been with me ever since: *What's wrong is always available, but so is what's right.*

BAM!

This hit me like a punch to the belly. I sat up, rummaged around for pen and paper and wrote it down. How true was that? I'd been watching the news and seeing misery, but there was lots of great stuff going on in the world too. I'd been bemoaning how hard I worked, but I was in the wonderful position of working for myself and had full choice as to whether I took a day off or not. Hell, I even got paid to exercise – what a bonus!

When I look back at my life, this one moment on my timeline is clearly a life changing point. From here forwards my desire to become a better, happier version of myself was conceived and realised.

It changed my thinking. Completely. That's what I want for you, too.

If you are always talking to yourself about how dire things are, about the person you work with being a pain, how the kids driving you mad, that your husband doesn't realise how hard you work, how heavy you are, how the scales don't move each morning, how you'd be so much happier if you could lose the last 3 lbs, it's time to stop. If you had to listen to your neighbour or colleague or sister talking to you all day about how rubbish their life was, you'd find a reason to leave the conversation.

It's time to find a new narrative.

I want you to think about the conversation you have with

yourself each and every day. It probably starts before you even get out of bed.

For example:

- Ugh, it's early
- I'm so tired
- I don't want to get up
- I hate my job
- Why can't the kids give me a few minutes?
- Is my belly big this morning?
- Ooh, I feel thin today.

As you go to the bathroom, you'll likely be having an ongoing conversation with yourself. If you step on the scales and it's not what you want to see, it can be the start of a bad day which produces more chatter in your head. The clothes you choose may be determined by your weight, as may how you treat your children, partner, colleagues. What's worse is that you probably don't even have a consistent rule for what 'bad' is. One day not losing any weight is bad; the next time only losing a pound is bad, and gaining a pound is terrible.

In some research I did amongst my clients and peers, 79% of people who weighed themselves would be negatively affected when they saw what the scales said. This is a lot of people wandering around unhappy because of a number.

On the days when the result is in your favour, it's a good day.

You dress and put your make-up on confidently, walk tall, smile more, have a happy air. And yet what defines good? It may be that you ate a takeaway last night and lost a pound overnight; it may be that you went away for the weekend with the girls, consumed a lot of wine and you've only put on a pound.

All these ridiculous ideas we come up with to justify whether we're the right weight are crazy. We make up the rules to suit us. And they are all random and unjustified, based on whatever applies to us at that time.

Take some time to consider what is going on in your head before you even get into the shower. What you're saying to yourself and thinking about yourself is a constant noise. It's more persistent than a toddler wanting a biscuit and not at all nice or kind.

It's a well reported fact that we get what we focus on, so if you focus on all the crappy bits in your life, you'll get more of them. If you focus on the nicer side, you'll get more of that too.

We all know someone who says things like 'It always happens to me' or 'Just my luck' when something goes wrong. Their expectation is leading them to look for how things have gone wrong. If we then think about the Tony Robbins quotation, something may have gone wrong a bit, but there will be lots of other things around it that have gone right.

Many people are sleepwalking in a bubble of bleak thinking so much that they have become blind to the good and only see the bad, the wrong and the lack. How about we change the narrative? We are going to talk to ourselves anyway. So, we may as well make it nice stuff.

How would you like to be spoken to? How would you speak to someone you really loved? If you can start your morning with these thoughts, you're halfway there:

- I'm going to have a great day today

- I could do with some energy, let's get up and get started

- Work may be a challenge today, so what can I do to get through it?

- The children are up early, so I'm going to give them a hug, make them a drink, talk to them about their day

- My belly feels a bit delicate today, I'll make sure I have a light/healthy breakfast.

You may have noticed there's not a hint of how much you weigh on this list. That's because in your new life, you won't need the scales. Yep, I said it. There is a life beyond the scales, trust me! But we'll get to that in Part Three.

Chapter Four

What Am I Willing to Change?

Accepting that you need to change and being willing to change are two very different things. You can accept that you may need to make changes to your lifestyle to get the results you want. Are you willing to make these changes not only for the duration of the transformation, but also once you get there?

Because of our access to social media, the perception of a perfect lifestyle, a perfect body, a perfect family is laid out for all to see. Yet we never see what happens to achieve that perfect lifestyle, perfect body or perfect family, let alone maintain it. If we knew what it took to maintain the look we so desire, we may not be so quick to wish we had it all.

This constant presentation of perfection taunts us that life will be like this all the time. Every day we'll look like a fitness model or be sitting by our pool because the online business churns out money without us doing any work for it.

I have a friend who, when I first met her, was a keen open water swimmer. She had swum the channel on her own a couple of times, and in teams had swum the length of Scottish lochs in very cool conditions. When you're in the open water for as long as she was, you need a layer of fat on you to keep you warm. So her normal physique then was very fit and toned, but slightly bulky to give her the padding for warmth.

Not one to think the extreme swimming was enough of a challenge, she then moved into another swimming costume hobby and took up body-building. She'd not done anything like this before, but finding out that she really liked it, she faced her fear and entered a competition.

Body-building is about lowering your body fat as far as possible to enhance and show your muscle form. My friend got her diet and nutrition right, her training right, accepted the fake tan and glittery bikini ways of the industry, and within two years had won an international award for body-building in America.

This was an example of both getting what she focussed on and making significant changes to her lifestyle to get her result. Her training regime was intense. Over a thirty week preparation phase before competition season, she'd train with weights four to six times a week and complete up to two cardio sessions a day, depending on her progress.

She was precise about her nutrition and it was highly managed. She'd count her protein grammes, her carbohydrate grammes, consider where to get her fats from and drink a lot of water. There was definitely no room for a crafty cake and coffee with a mate whilst in training. She would plan her days around her training and her eating, avoiding breakfasts at network meetings or taking her cooked chicken and vegetables in a plastic box rather than eating what was on offer.

Body builders, like anyone who strives for perfection, are training for one moment in time when their preparation, their management of their carbohydrates, water and posing practice all come together. Once they have finished competition season, they don't maintain this state. In fact, it's not possible or healthy. They go into off season to soften and bulk up again.

Sometimes this is what it takes to get what we want. This is the behind the scenes side of a perfect result that we don't often see.

Consider what it takes to get the results that you may see on Instagram or Facebook or in magazines, and what it will take to stay there. Then ask yourself, 'Is that what I really want? Am I willing to change enough to achieve it?

Change is also going to have an impact on others. Whilst I am not suggesting that you should only do as others wish, it's worth realising that when you change your normal, reliable routine, like having wine with dinner or going out each day to get lunch, it will mess with your friends' and family's heads a little. They may feel uncomfortable with the new you, and sometimes may direct this discomfort at you in a derogatory or incredulous way to try and derail you from what you want.

You may have heard people say, 'Don't be boring, have a drink with me' or 'How long is this going on for then?' or 'You can't live like a rabbit for ever'. These comments are an expression of other people's fear that their connection with you is being eroded. In some cases, it may be the end of a friendship, but generally, if your sense of purpose and achievement and focus is strong enough, they will realise that you aren't budging. They can continue as they are, but you're not going to join them.

In my experience, when I choose not to drink or have pudding, the people around me follow suit. So, take a stand; help everyone out.

Towards the end of the book there is a short guide for your partner on how to be supportive. This can also be used with people you see a lot, who may, with all good intentions, try to bring you back to where you were when they were comfortable around you.

Case study – Frances Mitten

One of my clients – let's call her Frances Mitten – had been suffering with severe depression for six or seven years before we met. She'd moved from a corporate job to a part-time job as the depression worsened and her moods dropped more and more.

Even though she'd been a keen sports player at school, she was now inactive and her weight went up as she got more and more depressed. She became heavily reliant on anti-depressants and, at times, said she considered her life to be not worth living.

A friend suggested she come to see me, and with much courage she made contact and completed her first outdoor group fitness session in April 2014. She was incredibly nervous, felt uncomfortable, out of breath and anxious. I could see it in her; she didn't have to tell me. Over the forty-five minutes I encouraged her to do what she could, keep moving, even if just slowly and gently, and rest when necessary.

All through the session, she has since told me, her little voice was saying, 'This is terrible, I'm rubbish. I don't have to come back. I just need to get through these forty-five minutes and never set foot here again.'

But as she left at the end of the session and walked back to her car, she said she felt something most unusual. Her limbs were buzzing and pulsing, and she realised that she really felt alive for the first time in years.

Frances continued to come regularly and steadily. One day, some eight weeks after she started, we were walking back to our cars and she happened to mention that earlier that week, she realised that she'd forgotten to take her anti-depressants not just for one day, but for ten! After six years of constantly medicated moods. She was so worried about the sudden stopping that she went to her GP to ask her about it. Her GP said that she would monitor Frances to make sure that she coped well without them and was happy to keep her off them so long as she kept up the exercise and new approach to life.

Now I am *not* advocating that you just stop any medication. But when you accept that you need to change (Frances decided something needed to be different for her to feel different) and are willing to make the changes (Frances kept coming to the fitness sessions despite feeling that it was a challenge), something will change for you somehow, whether you plan it or not. Frances hadn't considered when or how she'd come of her medication, and yet she did.

As a follow up to this story, Frances is still medication free and has established her own cottage industry business. She still has highs and lows and sometimes very dark moods. But she feels differently about them now. She knows they will pass, she knows what to do to keep them manageable, and she knows that she is on the right long-term path for her.

Case study – Helen

Helen had a similar experience, but her focus became more about the foods she was eating to accompany her exercise. She had experienced a chronic and niggling back pain since she was a child, and as a woman in her mid-forties was resigned to the fact that she'd be forever visiting physiotherapists and chiropractors.

She came along to see me to keep a friend company at our group fitness sessions. Helen was really keen to improve her moods, weight and ultimately health with an improved diet, and we spoke about what she could do to change it. At first, this was tricky. She has three children who, at the time, were older teenagers and were part of the family dining routine.

Helen cleaned up her diet by removing some of the obvious choices and saw some small improvements. However, her back would flare up and stop her from exercising, and this would throw her back into a pattern of poor eating, low moods and inactivity.

After a year or so, Helen decided to tackle this head on by removing some foods (as I'll show you in Part Three) that have been shown to be inflammatory and damaging for some people. She saw quick wins, her weight started to shift, her moods lifted and her back became less of an issue. As a result she could exercise more and improve her results. It wasn't long before she said she was having a much better life. Because she was happier at home, all her relationships became happier.

To turn her health up another notch, Helen and I looked at her diet more closely. Her back was still causing her some problems and she felt it wasn't a structural problem, but something she could fix with a diet change. After some testing and tweaking and further questioning, Helen decided to opt for a grain free diet. This won't suit everyone, but this way of eating really suited her.

The weight dropped even more, her energy went up, and despite eating more than she ever had before, she changed her shape dramatically. The best bit? Her backache went.

Over the next few months, she allowed some of the old foods to slip back into her diet, but soon noticed a negative change in her shape, digestion, moods and back pain. So, she has realised that her lifestyle has to be significantly different from where it was four or five years ago if she wants to keep the results she now has.

If you are ready and willing to make the permanent changes necessary to get the results you want, then go for it. Go for it heart and soul. Trust that you can and will do it. However, if you don't think it's for you, it's not what you want and your enthusiasm is more 'meh' than 'yay!', then please let it go. You don't need the constant chatter in your head of an outdated dream you once had. Find a new one and work on that instead.

Ask and Analyse Summary

Let's pull everything together in one place to get you started.

- Take your journal and ask new, positive questions that require you to think of your answer. Use questions like 'How can I...?' or 'What can I do to...?'

- Ask new questions of the answers to find the real reason for this need to change

- Work out what your values and beliefs are around the hot topics that are causing you to feel like you are no longer you

- Create a top five list of values

- Write down the internal chatter you have each day and how you can change it

- On a scale of 1–10, how happy do you feel about your health and fitness most days?

- On a scale of 1–10, how happy do you feel about your body most days?

- On a scale of 1–10, how happy do you feel about your energy most days?

- On a scale of 1–10, how happy do you feel about your mental/emotional health most days?

- Decide if what you want to change is something you are prepared to do things differently for ever to achieve.

PART TWO

Decide and Do

Chapter Five

Where Do I Begin?

As we move into the next part of the process, it may seem that we're still in the question asking phase. You may be asking yourself, 'Can I change this?', 'Will I see results quickly?' or 'What will this cost me in time, money, or emotional energy?'

Like any cleaning up job, there is always more mess before there is order. The tough, dirty work is in the preparation rather than the doing, and I'm hopeful that, like a good decorating job, we've moved from clearing the room and throwing things away to getting ready to do some real work.

You may have seen, or even used, a Wheel of Life. This image has been used for a long time by life coaches as a way of helping people find some balance in their lives. I think it works well when we give truly honest answers. However, sometimes we can be flippant and not really consider where we are at each stage of life. And it's a bit fixed. Like a wheel.

I want to use a more positive visual image that will relate to the efforts we put in over time. I've taken the same topics, but moved the image from a wheel to buckets.

We can imagine a bucket being either empty or full of things that we have put in it. And we can imagine knowing what the things in the bucket are. So I want you to imagine a bucket as a receptacle of contentment for each area of your life.

The areas that I focus on are:

- Career/purpose – (if you are working, this is your job; if you are not working, this is your purpose or what gets you up each day)

- Finances – home and personal

- Health – fitness, exercise, well-being

- Love – your key relationship

- Family – your kith and kin

- Social/fun – your friends, holidays, free time

- Religion/spirituality – your values and belief systems

- Physical environment – anything that affects your personal space, your house, your room, your car, your community.

- Personal development – your opportunities to grow and improve.

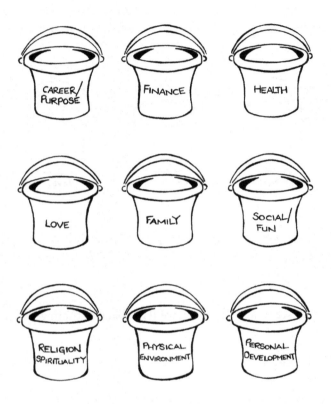

To identify how you are feeling in all of these areas of your life at the moment, fill the relevant bucket with how happy you are about each topic. Take some time and fill each bucket with whatever you like. You could just draw a line to reflect how full it is. You could imagine it with flowers in, or the things about that topic that make you feel happy. The fuller the bucket, the better off you are.

It may be that some of your buckets are full to overflowing.

Wonderful! One of my clients was in the rosy glow of planning her wedding, so her love bucket was full of big round hearts.

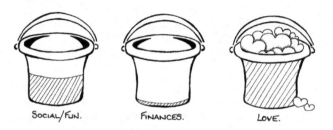

SOCIAL/FUN. FINANCES. LOVE.

This is your image. You need to know instantly how bountiful or lacking each one of your buckets is, so fill them in in a way that is right for you.

Keep these images for now; we'll get back to them very soon.

Life balance

Let's stop here for one moment and consider what it is that we are aiming for.

I believe that women today can be forgiven for thinking that they have every reason to be satisfied with their lot. They have a career, they may even be the principal earner. They have a family, opportunities to keep fit and healthy, places to travel to more easily and cheaply than ever before, and friends they can keep in contact with via the touch of a screen.

But they are often feeling overwhelmed and challenged and

unhappy as their personal experiences don't match what they see on social media, in films or magazines. They may have equality at work, but the reality is that in many cases they are also still managing the family, organising the social calendar, sorting out laundry, holidays, childcare, housework, meals and shopping. Whilst juggling being a wife/partner, mother, daughter and employee.

I know it's not like this for everyone. But it is like it for many of the women I meet who can't work out why they can't have it all *and* get the life balance they read about on Facebook and Twitter. Defining what life balance means to each individual is being sidelined in favour of a one-size-fits-all view.

Let me ask you a question.

Can you stand on one leg?

Can you stand on one leg and lean to one side with an arm reaching out?

Can you stand on one leg and lean to one side with an arm reaching out and your leg sticking out behind you, whilst your other arm reaches forwards?

Yes, you probably can.

Are you balanced? The first version was probably better than the third, but you will almost certainly be balanced.

And this, in my opinion, is like life. The times when we're lucky enough to be like the da Vinci *Vitruvian Man* with both feet planted firmly on the ground and both arms reaching out to the side are very few. Most of the time our balancing skills are put to good use with some wobbly moments, but we are still balancing.

So I want you to define what life balance means for you. Does it mean a split between work and home life? Does it mean work to live or live to work? Are your health and wealth buckets linked for you to have some calmness, balance and security?

Whatever life balance means for you at this stage in your life, write it down. Define it. Make a decision as to what is good enough for you to work towards. It doesn't need to be perfect, but it does need to resonate for you. If you don't know what you're aiming for, you'll never know if you've got there.

Bucket list

Let's go back to your virtual buckets. Now that you've defined where your life is at the moment, I want you to place them in order with fullest (happiest) first and emptiest, most barren last. As you look at your order, is it what you expected? Or are the buckets in a different order to how you imagined? Did you think that health would be at the bottom, but actually it's finances? Or were you expecting your family to be top and yet it's social?

I've found that it's common for the order of the buckets not to be as they were imagined. This a great first point in realising that if one of your chattering voices is about how heavy you are, or how fat you look, or how rubbish you are with food, it's because other more important problems in your life haven't been addressed or acknowledged. The bucket hasn't been filled.

As you look at your bucket list, decide which one, if improved, would make the biggest impact on your life right now. If you are stuck with the overwhelming thought that it's all of them, I want you break the thought process down to:

- Can I change this quickly?

- Can I see results quickly?

- What will it cost in time, money and emotional energy?

- Will the results fill my bucket?

For example, say you want to fix your environment bucket first and spruce your house up. Can you change this quickly? Maybe with tidying, but it will probably take longer with decorating.

Can you see results quickly? Nope, this will take time and will get worse before it gets better.

What will it cost in time, money and emotional energy? It will cost you in time (if you do it yourself), it will cost you financially to buy what you need, you may find it stressful. Will this fill your bucket? Yes, in the long term.

There are no right or wrong answers to supplying your buckets with more of what you love. However, quick wins will help you gain a feeling of success and momentum that will drive you towards working on the next one and the next one.

A journey of a thousand miles begins with a single step.

LAO TZU

So what are you going to do first? What one thing will give you the quickest win?

Sometimes the things that bug us the most actually take hardly any time to sort out at all. For example, if there's an annoying broken cupboard or drawer in the kitchen, fix it. Once that is done, you no longer have to fret about it. Your head will be calmer, you'll be calmer, and you'll no longer be having a ratty conversation with yourself.

Chapter Six

What Makes You Happy?

All of the strife we put ourselves through for not being slim enough, the right number on the scales, good enough or in the right job at some point comes to the realisation *I want to be happy.*

Many of the women I meet know that they're not quite right. They feel something is missing from their life; they think that they should be happy, but maybe they're not. They feel as though they have forgotten who they really are. Not knowing what would make it better, many don't even know what makes them happy any more. And all the time they're confusing this emotion with whether they were 9 stone 9 lb that morning or 9 stone 12 lb.

The women I meet and speak with want happiness, but don't

want to go for it in case someone calls them out on it. They don't want to be judged for doing something they love in case it makes them look a bit weird. And yet here's the thing: it actually makes them look stunningly beautiful.

When you do the thing that brings you complete cheek-rosying joy, makes you beam from ear to ear, brings tears of pure happiness to your eyes, you will shine from the inside out. And it's magic.

We've become trapped in a box of social expectation whilst surrounded by huge opportunity. Adults know more than ever that they can do what they want, when they want, and yet they don't. They are stifled by the routine, the 'What will so-and-so say?' and fear. It's time to break free. It's so worth it!

Your happy stuff

If you want to be happy, you need to know what makes you happy so that you will know when you get there. This is even more fraught with problems than finding the perfect diet because there is no perfect collection of things to make you happy. And this, I think, messes with people's heads.

I absolutely love a sunrise or a sunset. My Facebook page is a testament to this. They catch my breath and I look in awe at how stunning they are. It's not uncommon for me to stop the car and take photos of beautiful skies to capture the moment, the colours, the experience. But as I'm taking them, I'm crying.

Yes, they make me cry with joy, and yet some people I know barely see them. We're different; we tick differently.

I want you to find your happy stuff, the stuff you like. Open your brain to all the things that make you smile, cry with joy, take a deep, relaxing breath, pump you up or give you goose-bumps because you just know that they feel right.

EXERCISE. Take your journal and write out your bucket headings, one per page. Then underneath, write all the things that make you happy in each area.

Still not sure what makes you happy? Look at your phone – what photos are on there? Look at your Facebook page – what do you post and talk about?

Look at your Instagram feed – whom do you follow? What is already in each bucket that you could add more of?

Where's your favourite place? What's your favourite meal? Where's the happiest you've ever been? What music do you like? Is it live or recorded? What's your favourite colour, feeling, clothes, handbag, weather, restaurant? Do you like to be outside or inside, active or inactive?

What makes you cry? What takes your breath away? What do you want more of? When are you most relaxed?

You may not feel that you have much that makes you happy, but once you open this gate, you'll almost certainly have a whole herd of moments and things charging towards you. It's a lovely feeling. This list is constantly going to change. There will be times when what makes you happy may need to be left behind. That's OK, you'll still have the memory of it. But there will be plenty more things that you'll experience that you'd like more of. They are all part of you, so add them to your buckets.

I never knew how much I was going to adore Scotland until I went there. And after my first visit, I really wasn't convinced. It rained for six days of a seven-day holiday, and it wasn't until the last day that we even saw the mountains behind us as the sky was so close to the ground.

Why we even went back is a mystery. But I am so glad we did. My heart is in Scotland. We pass the sign on the M6 that says 'The Lakes' and I know I am nearly there. We pass the 'Welcome to Scotland' sign and I physically relax and feel peaceful.

I need more of that to make me happy. Luckily my husband agrees and we spend time there most years, sucking that all in. Perfect!

As you look at your list of things that make you smile, I want you to think about which of those things would make the quickest change to your life. Which is going to have the greatest impact on you if you take action on it immediately?

Take one or two things and go with them. Just start. It doesn't have to be perfect, because when we're happy, we don't care about perfect anyway. It will always be perfect to us when we're truly happy.

Your chemistry will change; your demeanour will change;

your skin tone, your eyes and your body language will all change. Instead of being weighed down by the dissatisfaction of not losing a pound overnight, you'll be doing something that gives you pleasure. You will shine. In fact, in my business we call it the glow. When we see someone change from grey and miserable to alive and happy, they really do glow from the inside out. It's beautiful and everyone comments on it.

Be the person who others are looking at and asking each other, 'What's she on?' It's called life.

Chapter Seven

Introducing the 1% Rule

In his book *The Compound Effect*, Darren Hardy describes an apocryphal fable about a father offering his two adult sons a choice. Would they take £1million today or wait, having 1p doubled each day for thirty days and taking the balance on day thirty-one. One son takes the £1 million immediately, thinking that he can make some shrewd investments and enjoy a lavish lifestyle, whilst the other son takes the penny that doubles in value each day.

As the weeks go by, the difference is marked. By the end of the first week, the first son is working on investing his money. The second son's inheritance stands at grand total of £0.64. After two weeks, the first son is enjoying his inheritance fully, whilst his brother is only worth a paltry £81.92.

In week three, the first son is still floating about on the giddiness of his windfall. By day twenty, his brother is at £5,242.88. By day twenty-eight, the second son has still not received a penny of his inheritance, but his balance is now £1,342,177.27. By day thirty it's £5,368,709.12, and on the day he receives his inheritance from his father, it is £10,737,418.20. A whopping 973% more than his brother who wanted instant gratification and ended up with a fraction of his windfall.

I love this story for two reasons. It reminds us that we do sometimes need to wait for the good stuff to happen. We need to wait for spring for flowers after winter. We need to wait for grapes to become wine. We need to wait for investments to grow. It also reminds us the satisfaction is in the process as much as the outcome. To get what we want, we need to be consistent, not perfect. Every day. Little and often.

I ask clients how they can make 1% difference to something they are trying to change. Mostly they dismiss it as being too much trouble. What's the point? The difference is too small to be worth the effort, and yet, as we see with the fable of the penny, starting with the smallest effort can lead to a huge result.

Case study – One red paperclip

A man, over the course of twelve months, traded a red paperclip for a house.

Kyle MacDonald took fourteen trades to move from something of low value to something of significant value to him. He didn't know from one trade to the next what he'd be receiving, but it had to be of increased value to him and move him towards his goal. All through his journey, no one lost out. Everyone benefited as what they received, they wanted. They valued it and it made them happy.

Here's Kyle's list of trades:

- Red paperclip
- Fish-shaped pen
- Hand sculpted doorknob
- Coleman camp stove with fuel
- Honda generator
- Empty keg and a neon Budweiser sign
- Ski-doo snowmobile
- Two person trip to British Columbia
- Traded one place for a box truck
- Recording contract with Metalworks, Mississauga
- Year's rent in Phoenix, Arizona
- One afternoon with Alice Cooper
- KISS motorised snow globe
- Role in a film
- Two storey farmhouse in Kipling, Saskatchewan.

A story of small, consistent incremental gains. Much like my 1% rule.

How to 1% your life

Do you know what 1% looks like?

If you are working on improving your finances, you could reduce your spending by 1% a month. Or increase your saving by 1% a month. It's tiny enough to be negligible, but if you do it consistently, without missing a beat even when it feels like it's not making any difference, you'll see one day that it has.

Average income in the UK at the time of publication is around £28,000 a year. If you save 1% of your income a month, it is £23.33 a month. After a year you have £280. Not a huge amount, but for less than £1 a day, you have £280 you wouldn't have otherwise had.

Keep that up, and apply it to any pay rises, birthday presents, unexpected refunds or cash windfalls, and your little pot of dosh will grows. And your life won't even have been affected.

What else can you apply this to?

The biggest barrier to people changing their ways is that they say they don't have enough of something. It may be that you feel your time is so stretched that you can't exercise or study or meditate or reflect or spend time listening to the children read. But 1% of a twenty-four-hour day is fourteen minutes.

How can you find fourteen minutes in your day to fit this in? Could you get up earlier? Spend less time on Facebook, watching television or Netflix? What impact would fourteen minutes' exercise (even walking) have on you if you did it every day?

I can tell you, because I did exactly that for 100 days in 2012. I changed shape on my legs and bum. I fitted in my clothes more easily and felt better. It set my day up and became my vitamin pill. Each day was not enough to effect a change on its own. But the compounding effect of the daily habit was huge. And it can be for you too.

What about study or self-development? What if you really want to learn a new hobby or skill for work? Could you read for fourteen minutes each day? Think of all the books you could read in a year if you did.

What if you are hoping to improve your health through the food you eat? Can you reduce 1% of your food intake each day?

I grant you this is a trickier one to manage, but could you drop the biscuit with the coffee, or cakes on Cake Friday in the office each week? Or could you have one less glass of wine at the weekend?

It's so small, it's almost 'Why even bother?', and this is the point. You want the change to be so tiny you don't notice it. But when you do it consistently enough, the effect will be huge.

In his book *The Slight Edge*, Jeff Olson says that the problem with small changes lies in that we don't see any immediate effect when we don't do it – so, we don't do it, brushing it aside, thinking it won't make a difference.

If you ate a cheeseburger and immediately
suffered a near-fatal heart attack, would you ever
go near a cheeseburger again? I doubt it.

JEFF OLSON

Moving to a 1% change rule is simple. If you're cutting back on booze, you can still have a drink with friends without them noticing you having one fewer than usual. If you want to be more active, you can add fourteen minutes' walking into each day. Some days you may do longer and that's a bonus – it doesn't mean you can miss a day, though. Continue with your 1% the next day. If you do miss a day for some reason – maybe you're ill – start up again as soon as you can. No guilt, no making up, no 'It's all ruined now'. It's not all ruined. Keep going and the effects will continue to compound and astound you.

We are surrounded by things that are quicker, more responsive and easier to get. So we have a misguided idea that everything can be achieved instantly. Not so. Medical school still takes seven years, flying to Australia from the UK still takes about twenty-two hours, and changing the shape or health of your body still takes regular, daily practice. So start now. If not now, when? Tomorrow will mean you get to where you want to be one day later.

Decide on your 1% today and do it!

Chapter Eight

Build Your Want Power

Does any of the following sound familiar?

You've decided that you want to lose weight and you've declared it to the family, your work colleagues and your friends, especially the one who always leads you off on a Prosecco fuelled evening. However, you don't want the family to suffer and so you keep buying them snacks. Crisps and chocolate dippers are around the kitchen as a constant reminder to you that you can't have them.

It's OK, you think, I can do this. I have strong willpower, of course I can avoid this stuff. It's all empty calories anyway.

Day one, you're strong. Day two, you're great, and by day three you think you have this sorted. But by day four, you rush out of the house in a hurry to get to a meeting without any breakfast. That's OK – you know that you can go without food for a few hours, so you'll manage.

When you get to the meeting there are pastries and biscuits laid out. You look, consider, but dutifully remind yourself of your iron willpower. *I can do this.*

By the coffee break, your belly is rumbling. The meeting is dragging and you're feeling low on energy from the early start. *One biscuit won't hurt, will it? Surely I can have one and not blow my effort.*

You sneak a biscuit at the break and feel a little guilty, but tell yourself it will be OK. However, this gives you a taste for food and your metabolism peps up and you're soon another biscuit and two pastries down in quick succession.

Sod it, I've done it again. I'm rubbish with food, I'll never succeed. I have no willpower.

Recognise this?

I'm going to ask you to forget about willpower. It's no more than an already stretched piece of elastic that has nowhere left to stretch to.

Working with willpower is a challenge at the best of times, and there will be occasions when you have to dig so deep that you hear yourself saying, 'Bugger it, you only live once' and downing a family sized box of Maltesers and a bottle of Pinot.

My challenge to you is to develop your *want* power.

Want power is your absolute reason for wanting a certain result. There are no questions, no excuses – you will do whatever it takes to get your want. If you aren't able to build a strong enough want power around your goal, then re-address your goal. Go back to Part One and ask yourself more questions about why it is so important to you. What will you have if you achieve this goal? What does it mean for your family, your career, you?

I am not being flippant here. You will work for what you absolutely want and believe in.

I am not sure where I got the phrase 'want power' from. I may have read it in another book, heard about it at an event or come up with myself in a moment of inspiration. But whichever way it appeared to me, it's been useful for the clients I work with.

Realising that the thing you think you want (e.g. the certain weight on the scales) isn't that important or isn't the real thing (actually you want to feel great each day) is so liberating. You can let go of the nagging thought that your willpower has let you down again. When you have want power, you know exactly what to do and how to get there and what compromises or 1% efforts you'll make to effect the change.

When did you last have a feeling of certainty about achieving something? A promotion? A pay rise? When did you last know that whatever happened, this was a done deal?

That's want power, and that's what we're going to work on – creating an emotion around a place that's so strong that it feels wrong if you're not there, and you'll do anything to find a way back to it.

See and feel

Conjure up a memory of when you had an amazing experience. It may have been your wedding day, or a great party, a holiday you loved, a place you discovered unexpectedly, a breathtaking view or a moment with your children that's etched in your heart.

Take a few minutes to close your eyes and bring that memory back to life. What happens? How does it make you feel to remember it? Do you get goose bumps or does your heart race?

Can you remember the feelings that led up to this event? Was it something you'd worked towards or something that took you by surprise?

Remembering how something that you loved made you feel is a great way to tap into your emotions around your want power. When you recreate these feelings, put them into a new project, goal, plan or bucket, you get the same energy and sense of purpose as before.

Let me share an example.

Remember my friend the body builder? She used this technique to win her World Title.

She knew she wanted to win and she knew what she wanted to look like to achieve this outcome. A note on her fridge reminded her every day what she was aiming for. She visualised that she had won, seeing herself on the stage with her trophy. Every time she trained, every time she ate, every time she slept, she had this image in her mind. She said that after a while, it became so real that she would get goosebumps.

Her brain was so used to the idea of her winning that it wasn't a stretch when she found herself actually winning the competition. That's the power of the mind.

I've done this too. I've done it to achieve work goals, personal goals and win raffles – yes, I really have! And I want the same for you. It comes down to one simple practice which can transform our lives.

It's the daily practice of visualisation and belief.

Imagine what it is you really want – the deep, dark answer to the why question – and see it with such clarity that you'll know what it looks like when you get there, because you've already experienced it in your mind. You're probably not even visualising the bigger goal here. You may be visualising the emotion behind the goal you want to reach.

It may be that you think you want to be a certain weight, but really you want to be at an event looking and feeling confident, happy and healthy. Or it may be that you want to compete in a sporting event and complete it well. The weight is not the goal; the outcome of the weight loss/gain is the goal.

Visualisation is a well-recognised and recommended skill that allows us to create the perfect outcome. I have a client who says she uses it for interviews. Before the interview, she finds out who's interviewing her (such is the power of LinkedIn and Facebook these days) so she has an idea of what they look like. She then goes through the interview in her mind over and over, imagining what questions they'll ask, how she'll answer them, how she'll come across, whether they'll find her amusing, capable and suitable or not.

She says it works successfully for her in making sure that she is confident before the interview even goes ahead. It works so well, in fact, that when I was chatting to her, she had won three jobs in quick succession.

It's used by sportsmen and athletes. The swimmer Michael Phelps was encouraged to use it from his early swimming days. His coach Bob Bowman instructed him to 'watch the videotape' each night and morning. This was a process where Phelps would go over each race, swimming turn, stroke, start and finish in his mind twice daily. He mentally knew every race, every possible outcome and how he'd handle it. I think we can all agree that paid off.

It's used for prisoners and offenders. In his book about the re-wiring of the brain *The New Psycho-Cybernetics*, Maxwell Maltz talks of how prisoners were encouraged to draw their visualisations and how it worked in reducing re-offending.

You may think that you're not a good visualiser or that you don't properly 'see' what it is you want. That's OK. There is no perfect way here. But if I ask you to imagine your best friend's face or the inside of a restaurant you last visited, I'm sure you can bring that to mind somehow. That's all it takes.

When I am placing my visual order with the future, I don't always see exactly what I want as though I am watching television. Rather it's a feeling; an awareness of what it feels and looks like. The stronger the feeling, the more aware I am that it will happen.

For other people, it may be a clear, strong image, or a series of sounds that they create to lay out exactly what they want in the way that they want it. This practice of showing the brain what to expect means, with enough repetition, that you'll tune into all the opportunities, people and events that will help you to achieve it.

Imagination alone won't get you what you want. You will need to take action and make decisions based on these desires. But you will be attuned to seeing opportunities when they appear because your brain now knows what it is you're looking for.

This may well already affect your state of being. If you step on your scales every morning and what you see dictates the state of your day, your focus is on that weight, that number, and how that makes you feel. Imagine if you could see yourself happy, feeling good in all situations, being active and healthy and successful whatever the scales say.

That's the image I want you to aim for. Starting today.

How to start the visualisation process

You can visualise anywhere – it's called daydreaming! But creating a habit around when you do it will allow you to build it up.

Firstly decide on how you'll know when your goal is complete. By this, I mean set your end point.

For example, as I go through the process of writing this book, I am using daily visualisation to get me to where I want to be. My end point could be when I've submitted the final manuscript to ReThink Press for editing. It could be when I've heard that it's gone to print. Or it could be me opening the door to the courier, signing for the box and reading the label to see it's for me and it's from ReThink Press. Feeling my heart pounding as I take the box into the kitchen then putting it on the counter, getting some scissors to slice across the tape, opening the lid flaps, moving any packaging to the side and pulling out the top copy to see my book for the first time. Giving it a smell and getting that new book whiff, then flicking through the pages to see what it looks like inside. Being aware of how new the pages feel. Checking the cover with my name on and the back page with the blurb. Showing my husband, smiling until my cheeks hurt, and probably crying and giving him a hug because I've achieved my goal.

Which one do you think I'm using? What's my end point?

You need to know when you've achieved what you want. What works for you? There is no right or wrong. If you were writing a book, it might be hearing that it's gone to print. That's absolutely fine. But create the feeling, the experience and the emotion around it.

Choose a regular time when you can be quiet and uninterrupted. Either first thing in the morning or last thing at night is a good time for me. Close your eyes and picture yourself in that place where you have already got whatever it is you are aiming for. You are at your finish point. Create it as though it's happening already.

Feel how you want to feel. See what you want to see. Put the people there you want to have around you. Wear the clothes you want to wear. Speak the words you'd want to say. Act as you'd want to act. Behave in the way you'd want to behave. Smell what you'd want to smell. Taste what you'd want to taste.

Do this for at least one minute a day, but stretch it to more if you can. The more you can soak your brain in feel-good, aspirational feelings, the more ready you'll be to pick up on all the people and things that will help you achieve what you want to achieve.

This isn't an intrusion on your time. You will be thinking and focussing anyway each day, so change what you think about to get a more favourable outcome. It may feel tough at first. But it's worth it. When you get this, your goals come to you more quickly than you ever thought possible, from world titles to books being published to being happy whatever the scales say.

A brief discussion on meditation

I've spent a lot of time talking about changing your thinking to improve how you feel each day. But there is as much benefit in taking time to clear the noise in your head with some simple meditative practice.

Taking time for yourself to think about what you want is key to good mental health and emotional well-being. Meditating, sitting and thinking, and being quiet are all essential in clearing the garbage of the mind and providing some clarity.

Meditation doesn't need to be a big, drawn out affair where you sit cross legged on a cushion and hum. You can do it whilst sitting at traffic lights, waiting in the doctor's surgery or travelling on the train. Just taking time to breathe and focus on right now and allow your thoughts to clear is good enough when starting out, and chances are you already do this. Making it regular daily practice, though, will bring some peace and clarity to your thinking.

If you are saying, 'I don't have time to meditate or visualise each day. I can't even get out the front door in the morning with a packed lunch, so when am I going to manage this?', the 100 Day Challenge in the final part of the book will guide you through it. But for now, know that taking time to stop and deliberately clear your mind can be very powerful in helping you cope with stressful situations each day.

Decide and Do Summary

Let's round this section up.

- Define what 'balance' is for you.
- Make a list of all your happy stuff. It could be a computer list or a vision board. Make it something you want to look at.
- Practise visualisation each day. Sow the seeds for a new internal conversation each day.

PART THREE
Consider and Change

Chapter Nine

Introducing Felt

Weighing themselves each day generally leaves people feeling either great or terrible. Either way, it's just a feeling. Now I am going to touch on four areas in your life that will help you feel happier each day without one mention of the scales. Changing how you approach these things will have the biggest impact on how you feel and your day to day happiness.

It's all about FELT – food, exercise, lifestyle, team.

F – Food

When your life revolves around what the scales say each day, there is almost certainly a diet/reward cycle going on that preoccupies you – 'What can I eat? What should I eat? Oh, I shouldn't have had that.'

I have clients who have said that they drive themselves mad with the constant internal chatter around food: 'What's next? What's healthy?' What they will have vs what they really want. They want to lose weight → they weigh themselves → they don't like number → they choose a diet → they think about all the other foods they'd rather have → they feel deprived → they work hard all week → they deserve a treat for putting up with their own crap. If you remember that you get what you focus on, you can see why they've found themselves in a cycle here.

Alongside changing how you think about yourself each day, I'm going to share with you some practices I've noticed around food and diet. I've used these myself, and with my clients over the years to varying degrees of success. It all depends on how dedicated people are to doing them.

Remember, this is neither a diet book nor a fully laid out nutrition book. However, I do want to share my own values and beliefs around food just as I share them with my clients to help them get the results they want, for ever.

Any diet works. It really does. It only stops working when you stop working at it, perhaps because it's boring or not a long-term fix or it's leaving you feeling worse than you did before you started. I know this because I've been there, and so have the clients I've met over the years.

From a small study I did, 30% of people gave up a diet within the first month, 46% of them citing that they felt deprived and ended up bingeing or didn't like being restricted around what they could or couldn't eat. There is no one perfect diet for everyone. Give yourself permission to stop following the same plan as your mate or your work colleague. There is so much individuality that will affect how your body functions, from the size of your stomach and liver to the quality of the cells in your digestive system, how much of your body weight is muscle compared to fat, what medication you take, how much sleep you get, whether your hormones are being artificially triggered or produced with medication, if you exercise a lot, are ill a lot, diet a lot. The list goes on.

Finding a way of eating that suits you, your lifestyle and your goals is one of the most important things you can do to have a happier day, every day. I've seen my clients change when they understand this.

My overriding principle for getting your food right is to go back to a place where you JERF each day. No, this isn't some tribal tradition. It's simple – just eat real food. Take it back to how it was before the rise of the food marketeer, making sure that each meal is as close to its natural source as possible.

What does that mean? It means porridge oats, not fast porridge in a pot. It means a home-made sandwich rather than a shop bought one that normally comes as part of a meal deal. It means a dinner of home-made chilli con carne and rice, not an 'Aren't I Good?' one from the chilled section. This one change alone will make a difference to how you feel.

Using fresh, real food will mean your body can work better and more easily. You'll have fewer illnesses, sleep better, manage your weight better and look sparkier. This is the best approach for a growing family, too. It's cost effective, as you can cook too much and freeze excess portions for healthier versions of a ready meal, and it doesn't have to take ages.

Within JERF there is another process that I use myself and share with my clients. I want you to start SWAPing your way to happiness every day.

s – Sugar

Cutting down on your sugar intake will have a huge impact on your mood, bloating, energy, clarity of thought, weight. After two days of cutting out sugar, your cravings for it will be reduced substantially; after one week, you will have more energy, sleep better and your cravings will be almost non-existent. After two weeks, you will have lost weight and bloating.

We are naturally inclined to eat sweet foods. We have sweet taste buds on our tongue and intuitively hunt down sweet foods because they give us quick energy when we are flagging. However, nothing in nature is as sweet as some of the foods that have become part of our diet today. You can re-educate your taste buds and find yourself saying 'Oh, it's not how I remember it' after some time off the white stuff.

I've run 30 Day Sugar Free challenges for people and they all say that they have great results. But if they should have 'just one' cake on Friday in the office, it sparks a cycle of a sugary food binge. Sugar really is addictive – just ask Google and you'll get an array of research papers citing it as exactly the same as a drug addiction. So it's not surprising that some people panic about giving it up, justifying their sugar intake with 'You only live once' or 'What's life about if you can't have chocolate?' And I am not saying that you'll never have it again, but be aware of how it affects you. Giving yourself a chance to reset your sweet tooth will allow you to have a choice about how you deal with sugar in the future.

During one of my challenges, I asked my clients what experiences they'd had after three weeks – good or bad? Here's one I want to share with you.

'I noticed some positive differences with less bloating, better digestion and more energy. I also loved feeling hungry for my meals as I wasn't snacking constantly. I was doing great until Tuesday last week when I gave in to temptation. I've added more sugar each day as I've craved more and more. The impact is that my clothes are tighter and I'm more grumpy and tired. I want to stop eating sugar again. So that's why I'm telling you all. Tomorrow I'm back on the challenge.'

Could you cut sugar out of your diet? At the end of the book, my 100 Day Challenge will give you some more information about how to achieve this simply.

W – Wheat and gluten

Whole books have been written on the impact of our growing appetite for wheat based foods and the associated gluten related conditions. If you are interested in the workings of this and why I feel so strongly about it (it's not just about disease, but Alzheimer's, depression and anxiety too), please check out the books I refer to in the resources section.

Reducing your wheat and gluten intake will have a positive impact on your emotional and physical health. But like sugar, it can raise a level of anxiety all of its own when you consider removing it from your diet. So my advice would be to cut down first of all. Eat fewer bread products, wraps and crackers. Choose vegetables over pasta and eggs over breakfast cereals.

Gluten is a protein that's found in some grains, including wheat, rye, barley, spelt, amaranth, semolina, bulgur wheat, couscous, and all the foods that are made from them. It doesn't include corn, rice, millet, oats, potatoes, quinoa, teff, tapioca, buckwheat or flours from nuts or pulses.

You don't need to be a coeliac to benefit from cutting gluten down or even out of your diet completely. Do it for a while to see how it affects you. In my experience, people who reduce the consumption of gluten substantially improve their digestion and bowel habits, and their memory – they are less foggy in their thinking.

Case study – The amazing results of going gluten free

I met a lady who for twenty-seven years had been pretty much imprisoned in her own home because of the effects of irritable bowel syndrome. She stopped exercising, going out with friends and doing all the things she loved. Over the course of a few years, she put on a couple of stone in weight and got so low she started to take anti-depressants. Very unhappy, she made appointments with doctors and consultants who couldn't find what was wrong with her.

When we met, I went through her history and asked her all

sorts of questions. When she mentioned her IBS problem, how it was stopping her from doing anything and the direct impact that was having on her young son, I asked if she'd ever been advised to given up gluten. She hadn't.

After more questioning, I suggested she gave it up for a month to see if it made any difference. She started straight away, and within three days was reporting that all was well in the bathroom. Twenty-seven years of being troubled with a daily dodgy belly, she found it all gone after three days of removing gluten. She lost a lot of bloating, her moods rose rapidly and she was able to come off her anti-depressants within about six weeks of starting her new lifestyle.

Did she get to the magic weight? No. Is she anywhere near it? No. Does her life feel better now? Yes. Is she a happier person? Hell, yes!

If you've got any undiagnosed digestive issues, from constipation to violent diarrhoea, or suffer from mental fogginess or itchy skin complaints, consider going gluten free for four weeks. I think you'll be amazed by what you'll find. If you are at all in doubt, please consult with a qualified nutritionist who can advise and/or test you.

Please don't be concerned about 'missing a food group'. Many people are coeliac and don't each gluten foods, and they are thriving. Many choose not to eat it because it makes them feel bloated and uncomfortable, and they are thriving too. Your diet actually becomes bigger when you ditch the gluten. It's all too easy to reach for the bread when you're hungry, but going gluten free makes you think a bit more widely.

As we go into the 100 Day Challenge in Part Five, I'll guide you to cut gluten out of your diet simply and healthily.

A – Alcohol

In my opinion, alcohol is to our generation what cigarettes were to my parents' generation. I am not anti-alcohol, but I see more and more people using it as their treat when things go well, or badly. Countless social media profile pictures show people drinking like photos used to show people smoking. It's become the cool thing to do.

If you're struggling with managing your weight, consider your alcohol consumption. For a start, the calories in alcohol need to be stored somewhere. If you are drinking half a bottle of wine a night, that's around 200–300 calories. If you've had your dinner and were offered another meal containing 200–300 calories, chances are you'd say no.

It has been shown that snacking increases when alcohol is involved, thus increasing the calories taken in even more. People who drink alcohol eat more than they would on booze-free nights.

Alcohol is disruptive of sleep. Even if you get to sleep quickly after a glass or two, the quality of the sleep is disturbed. It's also worth bearing in mind that if you've had a particularly boozy night, you'll still be over the limit in the morning.

I see many people, women mostly, justifying their drinking as a treat for life being terrible: 'Work sucks'; 'The traffic was terrible'; 'The kids have driven me to it'; 'You need a treat once in a while', or because life is great: 'Yay! got a promotion'; 'Home early, is it too soon to open the wine?'; 'The kids did so well in their reports #proudmummy'; 'Life is good, you need a treat once in while', or socially: 'Prosecco night, ladies'; 'Ooh, gin advent calendar, that's for me'. But the damaging effects of too much alcohol are unseen and life threatening.

I read an article once that said, 'When you say "I don't have an alcohol problem, I can give up whenever I want to", you already have a problem.' If you're looking at your mates doing Sober October or Dry January and thinking *Hell, no*, consider why you need to have a drink as often as you do.

I set myself a goal during the writing of this book. To get it written in the time-frame I'd set myself, I would get up earlier each day and write for an hour. My sleep would have to be in order as I already work long days and writing would add to them.

If I wanted to get great sleep, I could not drink in the evening. Even a glass would have me waking up early, sweating into my pillow, so I chose not to drink at all until my book was finished and sent to the printers.

Despite the stresses of the week and the habit of having a drink whilst making dinner at the weekend, I've done it without difficulty. Once my focus was on finishing the book, the idea of wine became unnecessary. I don't need it as a treat – the book going to print is the treat.

In the 100 Day Challenge section, I'll share with you how

the healthiest, happiest centenarians in the world have got to their ripe old age whilst still drinking, and you can too.

P – Processed foods

The P of SWAP is processed food. If you want to feel happy every day, eat better quality food.

If this is a new concept to you then take it gradually and slowly – remember the 1% rule. Ask yourself, 'What can I change today to add more fresh into my diet?' However you do this needs to be right for you and your family, fitting in with your way of living. Create a lifestyle that is easy to manage at home, work, on holiday and travelling. Remember there is no 'one-size-fits-all' solution, but I will give you some tips in Part Five.

If you were only going to do one of the SWAP suggestions, I would suggest this would be it. It includes both S and W to some extent, too.

Now you've got an idea as to how you can feel better every day by changing your food. If you do this the majority of the time, the likelihood is you will want to lapse into your old ways less and less, and if you do find yourself eating like you used to, you'll notice because you'll feel a bit uncomfortable or hungover. Your new way of living will be the better way, helping you feel happy every day.

F – food, we've done. Look back at your buckets. Is health one that needs addressing? If so, food is almost certainly going to be a part of that, so find your way and make it work.

However, there are some more aspects which will lift you up to feeling so great that your weighing scales will wonder where you've gone.

E – Exercise

There was never going to be a book about how to feel happy every day that didn't mention exercise somewhere.

I am a Personal Fitness Trainer by profession, it's in my blood. However – and this is important – I don't love exercise. I am not the type of trainer who has ripped muscles, does my own workouts to blackout and gets a buzz from going for the burn. I know lots of people who get their adrenaline high from exercise and that's absolutely great – if you are there, keep it up. But it's not how I feel, and you don't have to either.

Liking the results exercise gives you will keep you consistent, and that's what I get from it. I know that when I work out, I've done something positive for my body. My brain will function better that day and my mood will be lifted. Working out regularly keeps my digestion functioning well and regulates a sluggish appetite. It makes my skin glow, my muscles look more toned and clothes fit better.

If you aren't keen to exercise much, find your reason to do it. Is it to be healthy for your children? Is it to be a good role model for your children? Does it regulate your mood? Is it your 'me time'? Do you use it to de-stress or train for an event or wear your clothes comfortably? Is to do good for others by fundraising? Find a good reason that's true to your values because there will be times when you have to remind yourself why you're doing it.

If you have an aversion to exercise or sweating or aching, it may be that some of your early values and beliefs came from someone who didn't much like it either. Did you hear that girls shouldn't sweat? Or men won't like ladies with muscles? Was sport encouraged for the men in your family, whereas music and art were for the girls? Did your mum not like to exercise? Were you told at school you were too tall to be a gymnast? Too big to be a swimmer, like I was?

If you have some beliefs around exercise and your physicality, look into your past to see where they came from, then ask yourself if they are really true. Do you now believe them? See whether you can come to a place of peace within you that would allow you to be more active.

Remember the 1% rule – 1% more exercise is fourteen minutes a day when you start from nothing. Can you walk for fourteen minutes a day every day? Chances are you can, and when you do, you will feel amazing very quickly.

Whilst we're still on exercise, I want to add in one of my own needs that may be true for you. I need to be outside. I love it. Exercising outside, whether it's a walk, a run or a class, makes my day. It's not the exercise so much as being outside.

That is definitely my happy place. Find yours.

L Lifestyle

The habits you have around aspects of your life will affect how you feel each day. If you're gauging your happiness around the number on the scales and yet have inconsistent sleep patterns, your tiredness will change how well you perceive what the scales say. Even when you don't think you're tired, the decisions you make around food, exercise, how to speak to someone, how much wine to drink and how much money you spend will be altered.

I think that the way we approach sleep in the twenty-first century is almost as damaging as how we approach alcohol. It's become cool to brag about how little sleep we get, for example via social media updates on how much someone can do in twenty-four hours. This isn't cool or amazing; it's damaging to their health. It affects their hormone production, their moods, their weight management (insufficient sleep will slow down a weight loss progress) and general joy of life.

Getting enough sleep will allow you to feel happier each day. Seven to eight hours is generally recommended as being a good amount, and taking that sleep from 22.30 onwards is regarded as being good to work with the natural rhythms of the production of the hormone cortisol. Keeping to the same sleep rhythm even at the weekend works best, with naps in the afternoon rather than a lie in if you need to top up.

When you get enough sleep, you look more alert and bright. This alone can save you a ton of money on eye creams and age defying moisturiser.

One of my clients was quite amazed at how an extra hour sleep a night, three times a week, impacted how she and her boyfriend got on. They didn't bicker any more, their home-life was calmer and life was easier.

Take a look at your buckets again, specifically those around lifestyle.

When you look at your buckets, it's easy to look at where they are lacking. This is human nature, but isn't always the most helpful approach. If our goal seems a long way off, we can feel overwhelmed about the size of the problem and think it's too big to deal with.

Here's another approach to consider – I'd much rather work with areas of my life that I am already happy with, because improving these will have a big impact on all of my buckets. For example, it may be that one of your emptier buckets is finances and money. When you think about how much more money you'd need to make things right or how much debt you want to pay off, it may feel quite depressing and unrealistic. However, if you are feeling pretty positive about your work, it would be more beneficial to put your focus into earning more money, perhaps by going for a promotion, because this will directly impact the finances bucket. If promotion isn't available, then create a plan to improve your finances by selling clutter or taking on a new job. Find a positive approach to a potentially negative situation.

If another of your concerns is that you aren't seeing enough of your children because you're working long hours, this will almost certainly affect the decisions you make. It may affect how you eat, through guilt or remorse or stress, your relationship with your partner or your children, or how you 'allow' yourself time out away from the house for social or exercise time.

Making one decision to be there for breakfast and school run two or three days a week may be enough of a change for you to feel happier. And remember that any situation you are in can and will change. Children grow up; jobs and responsibilities alter. We always have a choice.

I used to work every night as a fitness instructor and would leave the house around 17.30, getting home any time between 19.30 and 22.00. Constantly not having me around had an impact on one daughter's behaviour at school. I had to choose between a regular income and happiness that I'd done the right thing for our children.

I gave up a night a week so I could be around more. Our daughter sorted herself out, I got more work, and within eighteen months we were in a new routine. But at that moment, it was the right decision, and my anxiety around doing my best for our daughter disappeared.

T – Team

You are the average of the five people
you spend the most time with.

JIM ROHN

When I first read this line, I had a mini-epiphany. It made such sense that I started to apply the principle to other people I know, and sure enough, it rang true.

If you're really happy and positive, chances are you spend a lot of time with people like this. If you don't like exercise, chances are you're not spending much time with people who do, and if you have a dieting mindset, chances are you're spending a lot of time with people who talk about calories, low fat and weight loss.

This is not a criticism, it's a mere observation. Give it a go. Birds of a feather really do flock together. Which suggests that if you want something different, you need to flock off somewhere else and find a new bunch of birds to hang out with.

And it works.

I've taken part in several self-development and business growth groups that all inspired me to be a better version of me, and when I'm surrounded by people all striving for the same thing, it really helps me get there.

Which five people do you spend most of your time with? This could be in person or virtually. If you spend a lot of time on Facebook, certain contacts or groups could be taking a lot of your time and forming your opinion on things. Community groups can be very useful, but they can also be a forum for gossip and ranting.

Are you happy with the impact your five are having on you? Do you want to step out or step up and change some of their ways of thinking and being? Do you want to change your mindset so you don't find yourself behaving in a way that you don't like with people you don't have much in common with any more? Getting your team right is essential to this process.

Yes, happiness comes from within, and yes, being happy every day is an inside job. But it is a whole lot easier with people who get it. They know why you don't want cake; they understand that going for a walk at lunchtime is what you do; they embrace rather than sabotage your new efforts; they support you and help you to succeed. If you've not got that with your current crew, change your flock.

Unfollow whiners on Facebook. It doesn't mean you're not their friend any more, you just don't want to see them on social media, and this is OK. Stop watching the news. It's generally depressing and structured to drive an emotional response. I am not saying don't be interested, but having your emotions wrung out day after day is soul sucking.

I stopped watching the news back in 2014 and it really helped me to feel better each night as I went to bed. I get up and avoid the news on the radio, choosing now to pick up the main headlines when I want from a source I choose. People who watch it hour to hour or have a headline ticker on their computer screen are preoccupied with the state of the world and seem to be in permanent worry and anxiety. Remember what Tony Robbins said? 'What's wrong is always available, but so is what's right.'

Find people who are already doing what you want. Find your new brood. Find your good news. Make good news!

Consider and Change Summary

I've guided you through a few key topics here to get the ball rolling as to how you can ditch the scales and improve your mood. There are, however, other buckets that we haven't touched on that may be affecting how you feel each day.

You may have financial concerns or want a new job, or your environment may not be conducive to you having a pleasant feeling about where you live or work.

Please remember that I want you to see where you can have the biggest impact in your life in the quickest time-frame. So for now choose one thing to focus on, one thing to make 1% difference to each day. That one thing will impact on the other areas of your life, allowing you the opportunity to address them when the time is right.

Trust your instincts here. Choose one thing – it will be the right one.

PART FOUR
Go for It

Chapter Ten

How Do I Start?

This section is about getting it done.

It's all very well talking about what you're going to do and how great it will be, but nothing changes until something changes. In this section, before we go into the 100 Day Challenge, I'll show you when, how and why to do it.

The 100 Day Challenge wraps things up in a safe, achievable programme that gets you focussing on more than the scales to be happier, healthier and calmer, not just occasionally, but every day.

Your first question may be, 'When am I going to start?' It's very simple. Now. In fact, I'd go so far as to say that you've already started.

I begin most of my talks with the line, 'You don't need to believe a word I say, but you can't unhear what you've heard', and the same goes for this book. You may act on only one thing – that's fine by me. A recipe book may only give me one good meal that I use time and again. If this book gives you one idea that stops you from believing that how you show up each day is linked to the scales, then I will have achieved what I wanted.

So, what are you going to do from now?

Move the bathroom scales. This isn't a question; this is a statement.

Move them, hide them, get them out of sight. I am not suggesting you never weigh yourself again. Doing it occasionally, for curiosity, is fine. But weighing yourself weekly, daily or multiple times daily needs to stop.

One of my clients this week told me how her scales can vary by up to 5 lbs just by her getting off and on them again. How can the weight they display be anything but useless? Put the scales in a cupboard; make it hard to use them. We need to stop this rot.

Once the scales are out of the way, what positive things can you do each day? Here are some ideas that my clients came up with:

- Get to bed fifteen minutes earlier

- Eat an apple rather than a cereal bar

- Drink 500ml more water

- Walk for fifteen minutes at lunchtime

- Spend thirty minutes after work with my children

- Balance my bank statement each week so I know where my finances are.

Chose one task that will have a big impact on your life when you 1% it and do it from today.

Test and measure

Knowing that what you're doing is benefiting you is essential to it taking hold quickly. If your old approaches haven't worked, or they have worked but only short term, your new approaches have to be both successful and sustainable.

The very nature of the 1% rule suggests that results will be slow and steady, but consistency is key. So how can we enforce consistency in something that we're not immediately seeing the results of? How will you know that what you're doing, what you've visualised and changed your thoughts about, is working?

I'll tell you. You'll feel it. Others will notice it. The people you work with will comment that you look different; your family will function more smoothly; and your mind will be less cluttered with how much you weigh and more focussed on what you can do.

If you are a visual and logical soul who needs to know what's changed, then go back to four of the questions we asked in the 'Ask And Analyse Summary' and see how you can answer them now.

- On a scale of 1–10, how happy do you feel about your health and fitness most days?

- On a scale of 1–10, how happy do you feel about your body most days?

- On a scale of 1–10, how happy do you feel about your energy most days?

- On a scale of 1–10, how happy do you feel about your mental/emotional health most days?

Because you are making constant small changes, the 1% effect may take a little time to make an impact. If you are saving money, that may take some time to look significant. If you are adding a fourteen minute walk each day, you may want to see if the smaller trousers in your wardrobe fit yet. Rather than using your clothes or the scales, ask yourself questions: 'Do I feel better? Am I calmer? Am I sleeping better?' Feel good that you've got the habit, not bad because it's not happening quickly enough.

Reward and repeat

Do you remember star charts? We used them for our daughters when they were desperate for a pet. They moved up the chart for good behaviour and getting music practice done each day, and down the chart for messing about. It took them ages to get to a point where they'd earned a rabbit, but it worked.

It worked because it was visible. They were accountable for their behaviour and they could track their progress easily.

We need a star chart. I don't care whether it's a children's one you pick up at the local stationery shop or one you make yourself. Having a place where you can see what you've done, where you've come from and what progress you've made is massively useful for achievement.

You can add whatever you want in the things to measure, but note one very important thing. There is a reward at the end. As adults, we don't often reward ourselves in a way that makes us realise we've done a good job. This isn't about posting it all over social media to get a quick feel-good fix; it's about deciding at what stage you want to recognise your progress on your journey so you can give yourself a positive and fun reward in line with your values.

If you are working on a healthier lifestyle, going out on a chocolate binge isn't a good plan. But getting your feet pedicured could be. If you're working on getting your finances sorted, going for a weekend away could scupper your work. But taking a day off to walk along the beach on a weekday may be just what you need to feel great and refocus.

How often you plan a reward is up to you, but I think 100 days is a good time to wait to mark the progress you're going to make. It's a long enough duration, yet achievable as you see that you are progressing towards it.

A reward every week is too frequent, in my opinion. The definition of the word reward is:

A thing given in recognition of service, effort, or achievement.

OXFORD DICTIONARIES

There is an action associated with a reward. You have *earned* it.

The definition of the word treat is:

(*treat oneself*) Do or have something
that gives one great pleasure.

'Treat yourself – you can diet tomorrow.'

OXFORD DICTIONARIES

Not one reference to earning it. I think people have got the two confused.

If you live to the idea that a treat is something you deserve when things go wrong, on that basis you could create a life full of problems just to justify a daily treat. The very nature of treats is that they are infrequent, a surprise. Daily treats become normality.

What can you set up for yourself every three months or so that you will be motivated to work towards? If you don't achieve your goal, don't take the reward as commiseration. An action chart will focus you on what you want, not what you don't want, and what you need to do to achieve it. It also allows you to practise the 1% rule of doing something little and often. Because the change is so small, you may miss a day thinking it won't make a difference, but having a chart will keep you on track.

If you choose to, you can share your goal with someone who will hold you accountable. Accountability buddies are popular in business development groups, and you may have heard the term gym buddy, or buddy system when you joined a new group. It's great to have someone on your side from day one. Choose someone who understands what it's like to make changes, but will still hold you to yours. Your new flock will support you on this journey.

During the writing of this book, I had some accountability buddies who were writing books too. We set ourselves a goal of writing a certain number of words within four weeks, declared what we wanted our rewards to be and then set off on our individual writing challenges. Our rewards were varied – a spa day for one; a weekend away for another; a golf shot gadget; a meal out with the husband; a day at the coast (for me).

Yes, we did it. And we all shared photos of our reward days.

Switch your thinking, switch your attention to what you want to create, and this will take your attention away from the scales. Not weighing yourself each day will make you feel better, giving you a reason to get up and take action with a clear head. Working towards a goal you want is going to inspire you. Working towards a goal that you are achieving with others is even more exciting and challenging as you're all in it at the same time, accountable to each other.

Chapter Eleven

What Next?

Isn't it a wonderful thing that, as human beings, we can be forever evolving, changing and growing? Life is not static. We are never done as new experiences come along to challenge or support us.

Accepting where you are now as being the best place to be and looking forward to where you'd like to be, rather than dwelling on what could have been, is a good practice to get into. Put your focus into what you want out of your life – shape it.

Case study – forward looking

I had a client some years ago whom I met when she was eighty-nine. She wanted a regular massage, but in reality she wanted company. I went to see her for six years, first as a massage therapist, but ultimately as a friend and confidante.

Despite her lack of mobility, I was impressed by her persistent forward looking attitude to life. She was a keen gardener, and although she couldn't get, out she bought plants so she could look at them from her window. Aged ninety-three, she purchased a young black bamboo plant. When it arrived, it was very green, and I questioned her on the name.

'Oh no, dear!' she replied. 'It won't go black until it's at least three years old. I am really looking forward to it, I've never seen one before.'

I loved her attitude to life. Despite her pain and immobility, frustration with the care system and lack of family around her, she was forward focussed enough to think that she'd live long enough to see her bamboo turn black. She died when she was ninety-five, never having seen it, but never thinking she wouldn't.

We're moving into pastures new, towards a programme called the 100 Day Challenge.

Life will throw you some stuff that will challenge your resolve. You may even drop off for a day or three. Feeling bad some days is fine. It's normal; we all get it. We ebb and flow through life like the seasons – sometimes we bloom, and sometimes we're in a dormant state. What we're aiming for is a general feeling of happiness every day; a knowledge that even if it's a crappy day today, we're usually a happy and upbeat person who doesn't use how much we weigh as a stick to beat ourselves with.

Putting a low mood and a jump on the scales together will be dynamite, so please don't weigh yourself when you feel low. It won't end well. Even during the 100 Day Challenge.

How you deal with these tricky life situations is important. It takes time. It's taken me five years since my Tony Robbins moment to get to a point where I feel really quite happy and pleased with my life every day. Along the way I've had some pretty crappy lows and some amazing highs, but I have eventually found a path where the peaks and troughs are smoother and life has a nicer glow about it.

As you do the challenge, you'll soon realise that the glow is you and it's reflecting back from everything you look at.

If you have good thoughts they will shine out of your
face like sunbeams and you will always look lovely.

ROALD DAHL

Supportive partner guidelines

As I was in the planning phases of the book, I met with one of my friends to have a chat. As I was tentatively sharing with her what I was doing, she told me how, when she was pregnant, she read a book that had a section in the back for the father-to-be.

It was so handy to say to her partner, 'Look, you don't need to read the whole book, but read this. You'll understand what's going on.'

I thought it was a great idea, given that many of my clients say that their other half is the one who struggles the most with a new routine. This process is tough for them too. They will want to help you, so show them how.

I hope the following guidelines will make it easier for them, so now it's time hand the book over to the man in your life.

For the men

Hello, guys! Throughout this section, the terms wife and husband will be used to include partner or significant other.

I hope you find these guidelines useful. They have been compiled by women who have shared some of the ways their husbands and friends supported them as they went through a health and lifestyle change. They also include ways they wished their husbands had supported them.

I saw a quotation that said 'Happy wife, happy life', which could be attributed to a lot of people. It's even a bit tongue in cheek, given that if either partner in a relationship is unhappy it will bring the mood of the house down. But if you can both have an understanding of how you can help each other to react and behave during a significant lifestyle change, you'll be on your way to a more harmonious household for all. My own husband has always been a supportive soul.

Here are the guidelines straight from the horse's mouth.

Fill her up with anything that's good, whether it's good food, large glasses of water, good words or encouraging more sleep.

Be aware of any triggers that may be a danger zone for your wife as she is making her changes. It might be lack of sleep. It might be hunger as she adapts to a new diet. It might be a withdrawal effect from cutting some foods out. It could be lack of time and not being organised.

Respect her decision. Questioning her sanity or commenting in a disbelieving way can be counterproductive. It may have taken your wife quite a while to realise that she wants to change her ways, and she may feel vulnerable that she's shared it. Help her get to the first hurdle.

Get involved. Plan meals, or at least eat them! Talk to your partner to ask her how you can help and support.

Find out what her main goals are. You may want to join in with her so you can support each other on some of the journey.

Listen. Your partner may want to have someone to talk to on a regular basis. All you need to do is listen. She isn't looking for a comment or advice, just a gentle nudge to remind her why she wanted to make the change in the first place. Help her to see if the change is still valid for her.

Support her unconditionally. Comments such as 'Oh go on, just one won't hurt' or 'you're no fun any more' are not helpful. Waving chocolate under her nose or buying cakes and leaving them in sight is not good support and will send your partner into a mood that won't fill the house with good energy.

All of us have a limited amount of willpower. So give her reason to succeed. Make it easy for her to do well. When she does do well, be happy. We are all children inside. We want to be recognised and loved and told how well we're doing, so if you notice a positive change in your wife – tell her! Your home life will be way more pleasant if you do.

> **Client story – Happy moment**
>
> The best thing my husband did was make me stop and think, and he didn't even realise he had done anything. When I was getting ready for my fortieth birthday party, I was looking in the mirror, focussing only on my tummy and moaning on. If only I had lost half a stone, I would have felt much better in what I had on.
>
> He said, 'Do you think anyone coming tonight will even notice? They are coming to celebrate with you because they want to and love you.'
>
> Simple – I keep coming back to this thought on a daily basis.

For me, my husband's support meant him backing off, not questioning my reasons or generating constant dialogue about the virtues of various latest 'fads'.

What I didn't like to hear: 'Do you really want to be eating that?'; 'Aren't you supposed to be on a diet?'; 'I didn't know that was part of your plan!' All comments like these do is make me rebel and I find myself eating more of the offending item just to stick two fingers up at him.

Please don't put temptation in your wife's path. If there's a great, big chocolate cake in front of me and everyone is diving in, my willpower isn't quite finely tuned enough to cope just yet. Out of sight is definitely out of mind.

Chances are you are like the many husbands I hear about each week. You love your wife as she is, for who she is and what she's achieved. You are likely not aware of the size of her clothes, the cut of her hair or any new shoes she has on. But you will be acutely aware of her mood changes, unhappiness or quick frustrations that seem unfounded.

Your support will help her to a better place in these three areas. When it's working well, the changes in her will happen quickly, and whilst she may not notice them immediately, you will. One of my clients told me that even her children noticed how much nicer she was with them when she came home from work because she was looking after herself and her health better.

Go for It Summary

A simple summary of this section.

Get started – there is no need to wait!

Review the partner guidelines and see if there are any you could add that would help you and your partner on your happy-every-day journey.

PART FIVE

The 100 Day Challenge

Chapter Twelve

Introducing the Challenge

The 100 Day Challenge was conceived in 2012 soon after I had retired from teaching exercise. I'd been an aerobics instructor for ten years and had loved it. However, I'd had an agreement with myself that if I ever got to the point where I didn't want to go to a class and had to put on a false grin to be there, it was time to move on. It was unfair of me to be grumpy in front of people on their leisure time.

Over the years I applied this to dropping a class here and picking up another elsewhere. But one day in the August of 2012, I realised I'd more than peaked. I'd done it. I was done with sweating for a living. I was done with telling people how to squat properly and I was done with learning choreography.

I quit. This was such a liberating experience.

I soon realised that I'd pushed my tolerance too far for too long and quitting was exactly the right thing to do. However, I now had a dilemma. For ten years I'd been paid to keep fit. I was in shape and healthy by virtue of my work, but this stopped abruptly.

At first, I was really pleased not to have to exercise every day, but after about three weeks I realised this couldn't last. I needed to do something.

And so the 100 Day Fitness Challenge was born.

I decided to reverse engineer the New Year's Resolution and do 100 days of fitness leading up to New Year's Eve, rather than after it. I worked on the principle that I could end the year feeling better than most people and go straight into a New Year with vigour and enthusiasm.

I'm a simple soul and I like to know what to do and when, so for me the challenge had to be simple to execute – a challenge to complete, but possible nonetheless. It also had to generate a sense of satisfaction at the end, whilst keeping me in shape given my sudden drop in activity.

I decided on 100 burpees every day for 100 days. (If you don't know what a burpee is, Google it and you'll get millions of hits.) It ticked all my requirements and I knew that I would be very chuffed to have accomplished that come New Year's Eve.

I started on 23 September (100 days before the end of the year) and set about knocking the burpees out. I'd do them first thing each morning, outside in my garden. My personal rules were no missed days and all in one session (not fifty in the morning and fifty in the afternoon), but I could mix up how I did them. Some days I did 10x10, other days I did 5 × 20 or 4 × 25 (my preference), and once I did 100 burpees all in one go, but that was boring and slow. I could do 4 × 25 in under ten minutes (less than my 1% a day) and I quickly saw a change in my body shape and fitness.

I did it – 10,000 burpees over 100 days. It did feel great, I did feel like it had been a good practice in getting a job done, and it did change my shape and fitness with the consistency of doing it each day.

Since then I've done other 100 Day Challenges. I've completed 100 days grain free, 100 days running 5 km each day and 100 days being active each day.

I run a 100 Day Fitness Challenge each year from 23 September to 31 December and use social media to pull everyone together who wants to get involved. It's a great way to prove to yourself that you can achieve something when you have the support of others. It also impacts other areas of your life – you become more organised, feel more motivated and have a purpose.

This is what I'm going to help you with here.

My 100 Day Challenge for you is to move away from using the scales as a guide to how good a person you are and towards being happy every day. People have a right to feel good each day, happy most days, and confident and full of life. This isn't some entitlement; it's a normal state of being and I want it for you.

Shall we get started?

This is a fourteen-week programme. You can start when you like; you don't have to wait until a Monday or the first of the month or 1 January or 23 September. Decide to start and then do it.

I'll take you through each week slowly. This isn't a race; it's a process to make changes slowly (1% rule) so that you barely see them, but you know that you're doing the right thing. Some weeks will give you big wins quickly. Others will seem like not much has changed, but with consistency you will effect a change and feel better every day.

I am going to talk about mini-rewards for every four weeks or so. These mini-rewards are for work done to keep you focussed on the bigger reward at 100 days. Before we start, think of something small to be a nice reward every for weeks, and a bigger one for the completion of 100 days of the challenge.

Chapter Thirteen

Weeks One to Four

Days 1–7: Water and liquids

I am still amazed at how many people don't drink enough of the fluids that will benefit them. Tap water is great for sure, but so is hot water with lemon juice or mint leaves, fruit and herbal teas, fizzy water or still mineral water. You don't need to slug back the plain cold stuff if that doesn't suit you.

When you drink enough water, you lubricate all the membranes in the body that allow you to function properly. Do you wear contact lenses? Keeping your fluids up will keep your eyes healthy and your contacts comfortable. Constipated? Drinking enough fluids will allow your digestive system to pass waste through you more easily and comfortably. Tired all the time? Dehydration will leave you feeling groggy, headachy and tired.

> **Case study – Dry eyes**
>
> One of my clients, a junior school teacher, was struggling with itchy skin and dry eyes. Her eyes were causing her so many problems, she'd have to take her contact lenses out before the end of the day.
>
> During a similar programme to the 100 Day Challenge, I encouraged everyone to drink more water each day. Within six days of drinking 2 litres of water a day, my client found her eyes improved so much that her contacts were no longer uncomfortable. She hadn't been drinking enough at school because getting to the bathroom whilst she was teaching was impossible to do. But she found a way to get more fluid in and saw results immediately.

Each morning, drink one 300 ml glass of water or a mug of hot water and lemon. Drink one more glass before leaving the house for work, one before lunch, one mid-afternoon, one as soon as you get in from work and one around bed time. Any additional fruit or herb teas count towards your total, but be less inclined to count coffee towards your fluid intake.

At the end of the week, give it a grade (10 = easy/great, 1 = tough/no result). Mark out of ten how much extra effort it required. Mark out of ten how much better you feel already. Mark out of ten how happy you've felt this week. If you've not felt great, write down why. Was it the weather? People at work? Were you tired? Get a feel for what makes your week great, alright or terrible.

Days 8–14: Outside time

Great stuff! You've done a week and this is a good start. It was a small change, but I hope you saw some impact fairly quickly.

This week we're sticking with water, that's not going anywhere. But now we're adding in some outside time. This isn't exercise as such; it's about being outside, taking some time to breathe more deeply, get away from the conveniences and stresses of the modern day and just be.

When I did my very first 100 Day Challenge, I walked each morning. I got up and walked the smallest circular loop where I live, which took between eighteen and twenty minutes. It was so nice to be outside and be me – no phone, no music, no gadgets comparing my time or steps from one day to the next. Just me, sunrises, dog walkers and my thoughts.

I appreciate that it's not always going to be a simple fix if you have school runs and commutes to get in. However, are you able to fit in a walk at lunchtime or after work, maybe after dinner or before bed? There will be spots in your week when you can take fourteen minutes (1% of your day) to get outside and walk.

And this week I am not even asking for you to do it every day. (That would be nice, but let's be kind and start easily). I want you to get three walks in. And continue with the water each day.

At the end of the week give it a grade: (10 = easy/great 1 =

tough/no result). Mark out of ten how much extra effort it required. Mark out of ten how much better you feel already. Mark out of ten how happy you've felt this week. If you've not felt great, write down why.

Days 15–21: Plants

Nice work! You've made it through fourteen days of doing something different, but not too tricky. Let's introduce another simple challenge into the mix.

Your goal this week is to add more fresh vegetables, salad or fruit into your meals each day. If you currently have a sandwich for lunch and pasta and sauce for dinner, could you add in a side salad with one of those? If you have toast for breakfast, you can add in a piece of fruit as well. It's not about taking stuff out, it's about putting more stuff in.

Here's what one of my clients said as she worked through a 30 Day Challenge.

'On the 30 Day Challenge, I have found that I have gone to more effort to prepare tasty salads and vegetables. I say more effort, but only in terms of thinking as the cooking and prep are quick and simple once you get into the swing of it.'

And this is the point. Most of the time we think that cooking from fresh is time consuming, but it isn't. The preparation can be really therapeutic.

Before you start this week, take a few minutes to ask where

can you can add more vegetables, salad or fruit into your daily meals. Keep up with the fourteen minutes' walking – can you do four this week? Keep up with the daily water intake, too.

At the end of the week give it a grade: (10 = easy/great, 1 = tough/no result). Mark out of ten how much extra effort it required. Mark out of 10 how much better you feel already. Mark out ten how happy you've felt this week. If you've not felt great, write down why.

Days 22–28: Sleep

You've done twenty-one days – I am really pleased for you. You've increased your water intake, got some air on your skin, eaten more fresh vegetables each day and completed one fifth of the challenge.

Well done!

Time to start planning how you will mini-reward yourself at the end of the first four weeks. I'm not talking food or drink. How about an hour to read or go out with a friend for a walk, or get your nails done or spend time on your hobby? I love to cook, and even though the end result is eating, I take a lot of pleasure from taking the time to do our normal main meal rather than rushing with something I know I can knock together quickly.

This week we're introducing a new sleep habit. I've left this until week four because although it will have a really reward-ing impact on your life and how you feel, it's one that many people challenge and fight and find ways to get out of. But given that you've done three small changes and recorded how well they've worked, I'm introducing it now.

Like the other weeks, make these changes in a small way. If you know you go to bed too late, bring your bedtime forward by fourteen minutes (1% of your day). This will mean starting your end of day routine earlier. You probably have a pattern of getting up from the sofa, turning out the lights, turning off the TV, locking the doors, putting the cat out, checking the children, cleaning your face and teeth, checking Facebook…

Starting from the first day of week four, move your bum off the sofa a little sooner. Go to bed. Get some sleep and your day will feel less tough on the other side. Don't set yourself up for challenging days because you want to watch a television programme. It will be on catch up before you know it.

At the end of the week, give it a grade: (10 = easy/great, 1 = tough/no result). Mark out of ten how much extra effort it required. Mark out of 10 how much better you feel already. Mark out of ten how happy you've felt this week. If you've not felt great, write down why.

We should have some cumulative impact by now. Four weeks of more water – reflect on what's changed here. Better eyesight? More energy? Fewer headaches? Less hungry? Better digestion (more regular)?

Three weeks of walking three to four times a week. How's that feeling? What do you appreciate about it? How does it change your day?

Two weeks of eating more plants each day? Has that been easy or challenging? Has it offered more variety, more bulk to meals?

One week of a bit more sleep? Do you need to tweak this more or has that been enough for now?

Yay! Go and enjoy your reward – whatever it is. Let me know on Twitter or Facebook how you've rewarded yourself for a job well done so far.

Chapter Fourteen

Weeks Five to Eight

Days 29–35: Your environment

I'm sure it will come as no surprise to you that what you've done up to this point is to be continued. You may already have increased some challenges a little. But if any have dropped off or been put to one side, then please revisit and add them back in. They all make up the small parts of the 'feel happy every day' jigsaw.

This week is about your environment. The space you live in or work in.

If your environment is not to your liking then it's going to be hard to be happy there, and so I am going to introduce the ten minute tidy (TMT). Taking less than 1% of your day, the TMT is a blast of productivity.

You're not allowed to do any more than ten minutes. This is a spurt of effort, not a massive project.

Each day this week I want you do a TMT at your place of work or home. I am not going to tell you when, that's for you to decide, but set it as one of the things you're going to do. Start with a room or area that's really bugging you (the plastic tubs cupboard sprang to my mind then), splurge for ten minutes then stop and move on with your day.

If this part of your life is already in place, then consider what adding ten minutes to each day will improve. Reading with the children? Preparing the next day's meal? Reading a book?

Enjoy!

At the end of the week, give it a grade: (10 = easy/great, 1 = tough/no result). Mark out of ten how much extra effort it required. Mark out of 10 how much better you feel already. Mark out of ten how happy you've felt this week. If you've not felt great, write down why.

Days 36–42: Time out

This week I am going to give you nothing to do. For some, this may be the most difficult one to accomplish.

Taking time for contemplative meditation is one of the best things that any of us can do for ourselves. Meditation is always in the articles that list five things highly successful people do each day. It's been practised for hundreds of years and is a valuable part of our ability to cope, reason and be happy each day.

When I talk about this with clients, I can often see their defences go up with a dismissive, 'I don't need that.' And I really like to quote the old Zen saying, 'You should sit in meditation for twenty minutes a day. Unless you're too busy, then you should sit for an hour', because this is so true. The more we shun time out to do nothing, the more we need it.

There are many ways in which you can practise quiet meditation. There are YouTube guided meditations that are specific for providing a certain state change. Some last ten minutes and some last four hours. I think that the best advice I can give you is to listen to a few to make sure that the guiding voice doesn't grate with you.

I really like the app Headspace (https://www.headspace .com/). It's a great product, you can set the length of your practice, starting from ten minutes per day, and choose what to focus on (after your initial introduction period). The male narrator has an English accent and the meditation is not totally guided. There is lots of quiet space for you to practise clearing your brain.

I would encourage you to choose the same time each day to meditate to establish a pattern. It could be done for ten minutes after you get into bed before you go to sleep, or first thing in the morning before anyone else gets up. Or take yourself out of the office and do it at lunchtime.

This week I am going to ask you to do three ten-minute meditations. Put them in your diary. It seems contrary to spend time doing nothing when you've got lots to do. Trust me, it will make you more productive and focussed.

At the end of the week, give it a grade: (10 = easy/great, 1 = tough/no result). Mark out of ten how much extra effort it required. Mark out of 10 how much better you feel already. Mark out of ten how happy you've felt this week. If you've not felt great, write down why.

Days 43–49: Alcohol

Completing this week will get you to one day short of half way. This is a massive step and I am so pleased that you've come this far. Well done!

I hope you completed the three meditations. I may have waited until week six to introduce them to you, but it is one of the best practices you can employ to give you the internal strength to be self-assured and happy every day. This week I am going to ask you to up it to five meditations across seven days so that long term you're not worried about doing it every day. The effects will be tangible and you'll feel you have some control over it.

Until now we've been adding good stuff in, but now it's time to reduce. If you are a drinker of alcohol and you'd like to manage how much you drink, I'm going to encourage you to cut back by one glass of whatever your tipple is a week. If you're drinking each night, then have an alcohol-free night.

If you're drinking on Friday and Saturday only, cut back by one drink on one of those evenings.

Alcohol has become a crutch for many people as a way to unwind, celebrate, commiserate and socialise. When you go out, decide in advance what you'll drink instead of alcohol all night. Fizzy water with fruit in? Fruit juice? Planning will help you know what to do when the time comes, when you've decided to cut back but aren't sure what you'll order instead.

With regard to how alcohol affects long term health, I'd like to draw your attention to the Blue Zones (www.bluezones.com). These are the five areas on the planet where the largest number of healthy centenarians are found. Living to 100 is one thing, but living to 100 whilst still being active and healthy is another.

Some research was done to see what the Blue Zones had in common with each other and nine different things were identified. One of these concerned alcohol.

People in all Blue Zones (except Adventists) drink alcohol moderately and regularly. Moderate drinkers outlive non-drinkers. The trick is to drink one to two glasses per day (preferably Sardinian Cannonau wine), with friends and/or with food. And no, you can't save up all week and have fourteen drinks on Saturday.

HTTPS://WWW.BLUEZONES.COM/2016/11/POWER-9/

You can have a drink and be healthy, but only when it's moderate and regular.

A little note of warning here. If you have never drunk alcohol before, now is not the time to start. Being teetotal has other benefits that will outweigh a regular tipple.

At the end of the week, give it a grade: (10 = easy/great, 1 = tough/no result). Mark out of ten how much extra effort it required. Mark out of 10 how much better you feel already. Mark out of ten how happy you've felt this week. If you've not felt great, write down why.

Days 50–56: Reinforce good practice

Halfway is a grand stage to get to, and I know what this feels like. In fact, it can be mixed. Part of you may be saying, 'Woo yeah, look at what I've done', whilst the other part is saying, 'Oh God, I need to do that all again.' I felt like that on my 100 days of running 5km a day.

On the fiftieth day, I ran a local ParkRun (https://www .parkrun.org.uk/) with a friend who promised he'd get me around the course in under thirty minutes, my personal best time at that moment. He got me round in just over twenty-eight minutes and I remember being staggered that I could achieve that. From that day on, I never ran over thirty minutes again. The limiting belief that I couldn't do it had gone and I knocked the second fifty days off much more happily than I had the first fifty.

Plan a mini-reward for yourself at the end of these seven days. Maybe a night out with some mates or a day off to do something you want to do.

Where have you struggled with this challenge so far? What could you change that we've already put in place that would give you the desire to keep on going? What if you asked someone to buddy with you? Would that make you want to complete the challenge happily and eagerly and see how you could feel at the end of fifty more days?

Here are some suggestions:

- Drop all alcohol for fifty days

- Walk every day for twenty minutes minimum

- Drink 2.5 litres water every day

- Meditate for twenty minutes a day, every day

- Cut out all processed foods.

At the end of the week, give it a grade: (10 = easy/great, 1 = tough/no result). Mark out of ten how much extra effort it required. Mark out of 10 how much better you feel already. Mark out of ten how happy you've felt this week. If you've not felt great, write down why.

Then take a day of reward and celebration.

Chapter Fifteen

Weeks Nine to Twelve

Days 57–63: Freshen up your food

I hope by now the whole business of weighing yourself each day is less important. That doing the right things for you to feel good about yourself is moving you towards a more satisfied, happy approach to life.

Until this point I've made sure we've kept the changes easy to do, simple to fit in, yet powerful in their effect. From this week, the changes may need a little bit of planning and preparation, but once that's done, you'll be seeing and feeling the benefits quickly.

This week we're starting with the P from SWAP. I want you to remove processed foods from your intake. This includes things like ready-made meals, pre-made sandwiches, tinned soups and jars of sauces. It includes highly flavoured and coloured cereals, snacks and biscuits, shop made cakes, chocolate and sweets.

It can seem overwhelming thinking about all the things you can't have, so instead focus on what you can have. Cooking all things from fresh produce means that you can still have shepherd's pie, but a home-made one. You can still have porridge, but from raw oats rather than out of an instant oats packet.

As before, start with one area that will have a big impact. Cook dinner from scratch four days out of seven. As this gets easier, increase it to five, six then seven days.

Cooking from scratch works best when you plan which meals you'll have each week and get your shopping based on those meals. It doesn't matter how you stick to it, but knowing that you have the ingredients for fresh meals helps take the thought and stress and mindless quick eating away.

If you need some inspiration, visit http://fasttrack-fitcamp .co.uk/

At the end of the week, give it a grade: (10 = easy/great, 1 = tough/no result). Mark out of ten how much extra effort it required. Mark out of 10 how much better you feel already. Mark out of ten how happy you've felt this week. If you've not felt great, write down why.

Days 64–70: Sugar-free wannabe

What a few months!

By this week, you will be drinking more water, walking each day, eating more plants, getting to bed earlier, taking time to get stuff done with a Ten Minute Tidy, having time out to reflect and think for ten minutes, five days out of seven, reducing your alcohol intake gradually and cooking more meals from scratch using fresh ingredients. When you look back at it like this, you can see what you've done, the changes you've made and how it all links together to help you feel better each day. We've not mentioned weighing or calories, yet we've built some strong foundations from which to function each day.

This week I want to bring your attention to how much calmer and more focussed you'll be by removing sugar from your diet. This won't be something that you'll have to do consciously for ever if you don't want to, but whether you remove sugar or reduce it, you will see a significant difference in your energy, bloating, appetite regulation and cravings.

I encourage my clients to do a 30 Day Sugar Free Challenge every now and then so they realise 1) how much sugar is hidden even in the healthiest of diets and 2) how much their taste buds have been changed because of the over-sweetening of foods.

This week's challenge won't be too hard – you've started already with the reduction of processed foods, but this is a good next step to getting you feeling better about yourself each day. One of my clients even quipped, "This is the easiest diet ever – you don't have to worry about how much to eat of anything. Just avoid sugar."

You'll find many guidelines for this style of elimination diet, but I want you to succeed and know that it's still possible to eat some foods you like. So here's what I encourage my clients to do:

- Remove all sugar, artificial sweeteners, honey, maple syrups, agave syrups, date and rice nectar and treacle/molasses

- Remove all dried fruits for thirty days to retrain the taste buds

- Eat fresh fruit for sweetness – berries are best, sharp hard fruits next, and juicy fruits and bananas next. Aim for one to two portions a day

- Remove all sweets, chocolates (apart from 70% cocoa plus), cakes, biscuits, sauces, pickles, etc.

- Remove fizzy drinks, fruit juices, squashes, milkshakes, fizzy wine, white wine, mixers for spirits and beer to start with. Red wine on occasion is fine.

One of the challenges will be to what level do you take this? Should you throw out your new lovingly made dinner because the stock cubes have sugar in? No, please don't! Should you make a fuss when your cappuccino has sprinkles on top? No, but next time ask for it without.

Going sugar free has been one of the best things I've done. It has shown me how my appetite can be managed, how I can escape from thinking that I have a sweet tooth and how much sugar is in the foods we eat. It's also an excellent balancer of body shape and weight.

If it's this good, you may wonder why I've left it until now in the 100 Day Challenge. The reason for this is that I want you to establish a record of succeeding to start with. Adding in some water each day is way more achievable than thinking about cutting out the foods that have been a crutch for so long. Build your confidence muscle before we move into this category.

Here's what one of my clients wrote of her 30-Day Sugar Free journey:

> I can sum this up by saying it is well worth doing. It is a very realistic challenge so there's a good chance to succeed, and well worth it. I am no longer always hungry, which I was when topping myself up with bits of chocolate here and there, and I feel more calm, less anxious and more like a person in balance.

The first few days will be a little challenging, but planning and preparation, knowing where the danger zones are – meetings with biscuits, colleagues with birthdays – will help ease you through. And remember, you don't have to be perfect. If you cut back on what you'd normally have, you're already winning – and 1% better each day is good enough.

At the end of the week, give it a grade: (10 = easy/great, 1 =

tough/no result). Mark out of ten how much extra effort it required. Mark out of 10 how much better you feel already. Mark out of ten how happy you've felt this week. If you've not felt great, write down why.

Days 71–77: Exercise

I am going to introduce exercise to this week's plan. I've left it until week ten as I want you to feel good with what you're already doing.

You've been walking so you've not been inactive, but it's worth considering that activity that either stimulates your cardiovascular system or musculoskeletal system or both will improve not only your body shape and fitness, but your long term health. Each week I see something that tells me why we need to be more active. I have yet to be confronted with a condition that exercise would be detrimental to.

I want you to think of exercise you like to do. Please don't start going to badminton because your mate likes it and you get a free lift, but you dread it all week. Find your want power – want to exercise and feel good and get better at it whilst having fun.

This week you can use some of your walking time to go towards exercise. So if you fancy going for a run or trying paddle boarding at the weekend, give the walking a miss that day, but make sure you hop back into the rhythm whenever you don't have any activity planned.

Aim for one to two hours of exercise this week. This could be one or two exercise classes at the local gym, four thirty-minute jogs or two forty-minute swims – I'm sure you get the idea.

At the end of the week, give it a grade: (10 = easy/great, 1 = tough/no result). Mark out of ten how much extra effort it required. Mark out of 10 how much better you feel already. Mark out of ten how happy you've felt this week. If you've not felt great, write down why.

Days 78–84: Thoughts become things

You're a long way into your 100 Day Challenge, adding the 1% rule as you go along and giving yourself some focus beyond how much you weigh each day. You've not weighed yourself – have you?

Motivational author Louise Hay says, 'Thoughts become things' and she's right. I mentioned this back in Part Two. If you think sad thoughts, you'll feel sad. If you think happy thoughts, you'll feel good. This applies to what we want out of life too, and so this week I am going to encourage you to swap some old thoughts for new ones.

Before you start the week, decide what you'd like to focus on:

- Your long-term health?
- Your long-term appearance?
- Your dream home?
- Your dream job?

Decide on one of them and write down (it's important you do this bit) what it is you want to achieve. Start with the words 'I am so happy that...' and fill in the blanks as though what you want to achieve has already happened.

Remember Helen from a few chapters back? She was my client who rid herself of back pain and unhappiness through a change in diet and activity. She told me, 'I used to see myself as happy that I was strong, muscled and healthy.' She now is. She thought it, she did what she needed to do it and believed that it would happen.

Rather than thinking, *I don't like my legs*, change your thoughts to what you want to have/see and be. This is a seed that needs to be sown first thing in the morning, last thing at night and every time in between that you have a free non-thinking moment.

At the end of the week, give it a grade: (10 = easy/great, 1 = tough/no result). Mark out of ten how much extra effort it required. Mark out of 10 how much better you feel already. Mark out of ten how happy you've felt this week. If you've not felt great, write down why.

Chapter Sixteen

Weeks Thirteen and Fourteen

Days 85–91: What's your purpose?

How did last week go?

It can take some time to change a thought. Thinking's a habit much like everything else we do, so stick with it if you find yourself drifting off to old ways a few times. Place your new image in your mind and live there as though it is already true.

With two weeks to go, I hope you can see a new future ahead of you. A reason to get up each day and feel good whatever the weather, the news or latest soap scandal.

There are lots of books and articles about finding out what

our life purpose is. I know that many people start to question why they're here as they hit the age of forty. This week is to think about what your life is for. What would you like your purpose to be for the next few months? Do you want to look after your health so you feel better about yourself and open up new opportunities? Is it changing career and retraining? Is there something you've always wanted to do, like a part-time degree or learning new skill? Have you always had a yen for travel? For voluntary work? For writing children's stories? Learning to paint or sing or ice skate?

See if you can dig up something from deep within that speaks to you about what you want out of life. And being a great mother or wife is a perfectly fine purpose to have. Many women don't feel like they have achieved this, and making this your purpose will give you the self-confidence to know that it's the best thing for you right now. Let this play around in your head as you're driving about, making a meal or listening to music. Your purpose may come to you, it may not. But be prepared for it to appear out of nowhere.

At the end of the week, give it a grade: (10 = easy/great, 1 = tough/no result). Mark out of ten how much extra effort it required. Mark out of 10 how much better you feel already. Mark out of ten how happy you've felt this week. If you've not felt great, write down why.

Days 92–100: Social media holiday

Look! Day 100 is on the page. You've made it. You've taken a gradual step by step approach to moving towards a happier and healthier life. Even if you only did some of it, well done! It's more than you would have done if you'd not read this book.

A part of me wanted to leave this week as reflection, but actually I am going to give you one more task...

This week, I want you to go social media and news free. No newspapers, no TV news, no Facebook, Twitter, Instagram or Snapchat. Just exist as a person in the flesh, not a person behind a screen. It's OK not to know what's happening all the time.

Discover things you used to do. Listen to music, read a real book (not an e-book), craft stuff, work in the garden. Get used to not having to share your life with anyone and everyone, and not having to react to everything that's going on around you.

I think this is one of the most difficult tasks for many of us. We love to take photos and share, to check in and discuss. But people used to do all this without telling social media about it. It is so nice to be gadget free – maybe not every day, but a day or two a week.

At the end of the week, give it a grade: (10 = easy/great, 1 = tough/no result). Mark out of ten how much extra effort it required. Mark out of 10 how much better you feel already. Mark out of ten how happy you've felt this week. If you've not felt great, write down why.

Chapter Seventeen

Day 101 and Onwards

Oh my! One hundred days ago, you decided to start this journey with me.

I like a challenge that lasts 100 days. It's long enough for it to be concerted and definite. It's also long enough for you to have to focus on it, giving you a reason each day to work towards it. It allows the 1% rule to come into effect and have some impact. It's satisfying when you get to the end.

Ah, 'the end' – those magical words you may have been uttering to yourself over the last few months. 'At the end of this, I will...'

And there's the thing. There is no end to this. The 100 Day Challenge has been the start of a longer, more rewarding journey. A programme that keeps on giving the more you give to it.

All the changes you've discovered as you've gone along have been the accumulation of lots of little pieces of effort that, when added together, produce a happier, chirpier person. Someone who gets on with purpose each day, without having to weigh themselves first to check if they're worthy. So choose where you go from here.

How are your buckets looking now? Is there an area that needs some attention? Can you rework your week a little to put some focus there (1% it) to make the change, but not let it overwhelm you? What small thing could you do each day to move you towards a bucket that overflows with satisfaction and contentment?

I've started you off with what I think is a good foundation for feeling better from the inside out. Now you can look at where you are again and redefine how you can improve your outcome. Would a twenty minute meditation a few times a week be beneficial? Would two really hard workout sessions a week and walks on the other five be enough to keep you feeling good about your health? Would another fifteen to thirty minutes' sleep each night help you out?

Whatever you decide to do, keep going from Day 101. This is your pattern now, there's no need to stop. It's who you are and what you do. Look forward to doing the best you can in your thoughts, your food and how you move each day.

You know how you've done – you've done 100 days, so feel proud and pleased with that.

Please condemn your scales to the big scales graveyard. Yes, work on your health to feel better, move more easily, wear smaller clothes. Practise daily habits that leave you feeling good and happy. But don't let a certain number define your success. You will forever be chasing the dream.

To your very happy days.

I want to leave you with this story from Helen, one of my most successful clients, who told me where she was, where she's got to and what made her succeed.

Helen's story

People say it's boring eating healthily. I'll tell you what is boring:

- Being fat
- Feeling depressed
- Being bloated all the time
- Feeling exhausted
- Being paranoid
- Getting miserable about clothes not fitting
- Not wanting to go on sunny holidays
- Feeling self-conscious

- Thinking about your weight continuously.

I worried so much about being forty in the depressed, unfit and fat state I was in. I was in a cycle of weighing, punishing myself then feeling more depressed.

Even on days when I felt thinner, I'd weigh myself only to discover I was a little heavier than the day before. It would ruin my day, I'd panic and eat more of the things that were making me fat.

Weighing myself was having the opposite effect to what I really wanted and needed, so I decided I wasn't going to weigh myself like that any more. I also stopped trying to lose weight for events like weddings, weekends away and parties, etc. I realised it wasn't a race. It had to be a more long-term goal without the enormous amount of pressure.

I stopped treating unhealthy foods as a joke when I ate them. I knew it wasn't funny; it was a serious issue for me as I knew they'd make me sick. My health and happiness relied on me giving them up.

I had a vision of what I wanted my life to look like. It was to be happy, strong and healthy. I was already exercising and realised what foods were holding me back, so I stopped focussing on what I couldn't eat and my weight, and refocussed on what healthy, energising foods I could eat, and that I could make them tasty.

If I did eat something not so healthy, I refused to feel guilty as I knew it would be detrimental and probably make me want to jump on the scales. So, when I did have a blip, I got straight back on with healthy eating.

I made more thoughtful, slower choices about foods I didn't want to be eating. I would take a minute to think how I'd feel if I ate something, for example imagining leaving a café having eaten ice cream feeling guilty, fat, beaten and stupid for giving in. Then I'd imagine not having eaten it. I knew I'd feel strong – that I had the power over food, not it over me. Before I knew it, I was needing new clothes, people were telling me I'd lost weight, and best of all, I felt great!

Now I am nearly fifty and not the person I was at forty. I often think of the period around my fortieth birthday as being such an utter waste of time. However, it did me a favour. I wonder whether I'd be doing all the health and fitness stuff and feeling happy every day if things hadn't got so bad.

Closing Thought

I've worked with over 1,500 adults to help them get fitter, feel better and function well.

There was one special group of ten women. I did some work with them over a period of four months to help with their internal views of themselves as well as their health and fitness. They were all unhappy with their weight and shape, so we spent some time looking at values and resetting the belief that they weren't good enough.

I asked them a question: 'What one thing would you tell your daughter/friend/mum about how to be happy?'

And here's what they came up with.

- Don't get caught up in what other people think

- Spend time with the people who matter to you

- Love yourself as much as you did before you learned differently

- Happiness is the journey, not the destination

- Don't forget everyone else is winging it too

- Be kind to yourself first

- Live the life you want, not the life others tell you that you should be living

- You are in control of how good or bad each day is – how you react to situations defines your day

- Live in the moment

- Be thoughtful about yourself, others and your environment.

And not one mention of weight...

Resources

Self-improvement

You Can Heal Your Life, Louise Hay

The Slight Edge, Jeff Olson

Unleash the Power Within, Tony Robbins

Compound Effect, Darren Hardy

The New Psycho-Cybernetics, Maxwell Maltz

Food and health

The Blue Zones, Dan Buettner

Wheat Belly, William Davis

Grain Brain, Dr David Perlmutter

Brain Maker, Dr David Perlmutter

The Mood Cure, Julia Ross

Acknowledgements

There are always a lot of people involved in pulling a project together. I hope I don't miss anyone but I'd like to thank the following people for helping me along the way to the completion of my first book.

Thank you to Nia Wyn-Jones, Heidi Sandford and Natasha Kearslake for reading the the early version. I needed that incentive to get it written and handed to you all.

The KPI Dream Team, James Herbertson, James White, Emily Macpherson, Julia Kendrick and Michael Anderson for being the rocks from which this project was carved.

Daniel Priestley and Andrew Priestley at Dent who sowed

the seed of possibility that I could write a book, even if it was for just one person.

Thank you to Lucy McCarraher, Joe Gregory and the editing team at Rethink Press for their kind, timely and consistent approach to helping get a book out from a first-time author.

To Heidi Sandford aka Frances Mitten, for her illustrations of buckets.

Karen Burles, Kirsty Boswell, Vicki Judd, Laura Parsons, Porscha Davies and Emma Wade. My team of instructors at FastTrack Fit Camp for helping me out when I needed them to so I could get my words written.

To my loyal and health-conscious clients at FastTrack Fit Camp who have followed my blogs, answered my surveys, asked about progress and taken an interest in this project.

Finally, thanks go to my family for putting up with yet another idea for another project. To my daughters Laura and Sophie for making sure I got this finished and to Dale who has never once mentioned my weight or size in all our years together. Thank you.

The Author

Heidi has had an interest in health, fitness and food since she was 10 years old, when she moved directly from reading Enid Blyton's spiffing adventures to recipe books and health guides.

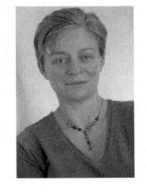

After a series of unexciting office jobs in her twenties, Heidi retrained as a Personal Trainer and Group Fitness Instructor in her thirties and discovered an industry that she felt at home in. Despite the improved fitness, her own weight and mood was erratic and she felt as though she was always trying to find an answer to what could make her better.

Following a slew of self-development courses, changing her diet multiple times a year and reading voraciously in the area of self improvement, Heidi found a way that gave her the confidence, satisfaction and balanced approach to her own health that she talks about today.

Heidi owns and runs FastTrack Fit Camp, a large independent bootcamp business helping people between 40 and 60 to feel better every day, regardless of their clothes size or weight. She is a respected speaker and facilitator of workshops in the areas of health, wellness and helping micro-businesses to have a healthy view of entrepreneurship.

Heidi lives in Wokingham, Berkshire in the south east of England and is married to Dale. They have two adult daughters, Laura and Sophie, who have adopted the 'happy every day' mantra and made it their own.

Heidi can be contacted at:
heidi@fasttrack-fitcamp.co.uk
Facebook: www.facebook.com/heidistrickers
Twitter: twitter.com/heidistrickers
Website: www.heidi.strickland-clark.co.uk

Lightning Source UK Ltd.
Milton Keynes UK
UKOW01f2354110917
309020UK00005B/197/P